Quality Management in Ambulatory Care

Patrice L. Spath, Editor

AHA books are published by American Hospital Publishing, Inc.,
an American Hospital Association company

Library of Congress Cataloging-in-Publication Data

Quality management in ambulatory care / Patrice L. Spath, editor.
      p.   cm.
  Includes bibliographical references.
  ISBN 1-55648-090-3 (pbk.)
  1. Ambulatory medical care—Quality control.   I. Spath, Patrice.
  [DNLM: 1. Ambulatory Care—organization & administration.
2. Ambulatory Care—standards.   3. Quality Assurance, Health Care—
organization & administration.   4. Quality Assurance, Health Care—
standards.   WX 205 Q15]
RA399.A1Q35   1992
362.1′068′5—dc20
DNLM/DLC
for Library of Congress   92-17698
                                                                      CIP

Catalog no. 169104

©1992 by American Hospital Publishing Inc.,
an American Hospital Association company

Printed in the USA

Text set in Palacio
4M—08/92—0321

Audrey Kaufman, Project Editor
Linda Conheady, Manuscript Editor
Teresa Cappetta-Kroger, Editorial Assistant
Marcia Bottoms, Managing Editor
Peggy DuMais, Production Coordinator
Cheryl Kusek, Cover Designer
Brian Schenk, Books Division Director

Contents

About the Editor

Patrice L. Spath is president of Brown-Spath and Associates, Portland, Oregon, which provides health care quality and resource management consulting and education. Previously, Ms. Spath was patient review systems coordinator at Meridian Park Hospital in Tualatin, Oregon. Ms. Spath is the editor of *Innovations in Health Care Quality Measurement*, which was published by AHPI in 1989.

Contributors

Pam Blackmore is vice-president of Schubert Associates, Sacramento, California, an organization that provides health care management consultation for health care organizations.

Susan Dahl, R.R.A., is the health systems development director for the California Rural Indian Health Board in Sacramento. She is also owner of a consulting firm, Contemporary Health Management Systems, in Sacramento.

Cathy Disch is an administrator in ambulatory services at the University of Texas, Medical Branch, Galveston.

Elizabeth C. Doherty, Ph.D., C.P.H.Q., is the liaison for regulatory agency activity in the quality improvement program at the University of Pittsburgh Medical Center, Pittsburgh, Pennsylvania.

Paul Frisch, J.D., C.A.E., is director of medical–legal affairs for the Oregon Medical Association in Portland and a consulting member of the patient safety/risk management subcommittee of the American Medical Association/Specialty Society Medical Liability Project.

Mary P. Jackson, R.N., is a Learning Center Resource nurse in the Department of Nursing Education, Development and Research, St. Luke's–Roosevelt Hospital Center, New York City. Prior to this position she was the quality assurance coordinator for ambulatory care, St. Luke's–Roosevelt Hospital Center, where she developed and implemented the Quality Assurance Program and monitoring tools for the hospital-based clinics. Her additional clinical background includes 20 years of emergency nursing, as well as pediatric and ambulatory care experience.

Priscilla Kibbee is president of Allds Associates, an organization in Wolcott, New York, that provides quality management consulting for health care organizations.

amples of implementation, and scoring guidelines. (A scoring guideline is a descriptive tool that is used to assist hospitals in their efforts to comply with Joint Commission standards and to determine degrees of compliance.) Scoring guidelines assist hospitals in preparing for accreditation surveys and were developed to reduce surveyor variation in the evaluation process.

A future component of the Agenda for Change is the development of an indicator-based performance system. (An indicator is a tool used to measure an organization's performance of functions, processes, and outcomes over time.) Monitoring indicators have been developed for obstetric and perioperative care. Trauma, oncology, and cardiovascular indicators will be added in 1995. Providers are being encouraged to develop indicators that are specific to each unique function of patient care.

NUTRITION CARE STANDARDS DEVELOPMENT

The first assignment for the interdisciplinary task force of physicians, nurses, dietitians, and pharmacists by the JCAHO staff was to identify the essential components of the nutrition care process. Nutrition care is defined by the JCAHO as "the intervention and counseling of individuals on appropriate nutrition intake by integrating information from the nutrition assessment with information on food and other sources of nutrients and meal preparation consistent with cultural background and socioeconomic status. A component of medical treatment, nutrition therapy includes enteral and parenteral nutrition." A flow diagram was developed by the task force to identify the nutrition care process (Figure 1). As a component of patient care, nutrition care consists of (1) screening, assessment, and reassessment;

(2) planning; (3) ordering; (4) preparing and distributing or administering; and (5) monitoring. The clinical algorithm[1] for the use of parenteral and enteral nutrition should be used as part of the assessment to determine the appropriate route for delivery of nutrition support.

Eight new standards have been defined to establish requirements for nutrition care to be provided to the patient (see chart below). None of the standards are unexpected; each defines a step in the process of providing nutrition care, as indicated in Figure 1.

NUTRITION CARE STANDARDS

TX.4 A plan for nutrition therapy is developed, and/or a prescription or order for food or a nutrition product(s) is provided for all patients as appropriate.

TX.4.1 For those patients determined to be at nutrition risk, an interdisciplinary plan for nutrition therapy is developed and revised, as appropriate to the patient's need.

TX.4.2 Authorized individuals prescribe or order food and nutrition products in a timely manner.

TX.4.3 Responsibility for preparing, storing, distributing, and administering food and nutrition products is defined and assigned.

TX.4.4 Food and nutrition products are distributed and administered in a safe, accurate, timely, and acceptable manner to the patient for whom they have been prescribed or ordered.

TX.4.5 Each patient is monitored for the nutrition's effectiveness and appropriateness.

TX.4.6 The organization has a functioning process for providing food and nutrition products when diets or diet schedules are altered.

TX.4.7 The organization has a functioning mechanism designed to standardize and communicate nutrition care approaches and processes throughout the organization.

All of the chapters in the sections on patient-focused functions relate to nutrition care providers. Thus all providers need to be familiar with and guided by the critical points for each of the standards in this section. Specific standards from each of the chapters in the section are presented.

Patient Rights and Organizational Ethics. The theme present in this section is consistent throughout the manual: patients or their families have the right to make decisions related to their access to care and to various treatments and their care should be provided with respect. More emphasis on the importance of assessing each individual's unique needs has been included in all of the standards. This includes adjusting care to meet patients' psychosocial, cultural, and spiritual needs, with treatment plans that are realistic and compatible with the resources of the patients and their community. Table 2 provides an example of the implementation of patients' rights for nutrition care providers.

Assessment of Patients. Within 24 hours after admission, the patient's history and physical examination must be completed or documented. The history and results of physical examinations that were obtained within 30 days before admission can be submitted for the medical record. Additional assessment must be made of the patient's physical, psychologic, and social status, and the need for assessing the patient's nutritional status must be determined. The suggested implementation of compliance with this standard is to have a nutrition planning process in place that includes screening. The JCAHO defines nutrition screening as "the process of identifying characteristics known to be associated with nutrition problems. Its purpose is

Beverley J. Moir was director of quality services at The Hospital for Sick Children in Toronto, Canada, during the development of this project. She is currently a health management consultant with CHCL Comprehensive Healthcare Consultants, Ltd., which is headquartered in Ottawa, Ontario. Her duties include managing and developing the company's Toronto office practice.

Emil F. Pascarelli, M.D., is director of ambulatory care at St. Luke's–Roosevelt Hospital Center, New York City.

Dewey C. Scheid, M.D., is clinical associate director of West Side Family Practice Center, Akron General Medical Center, Ohio; associate medical director of Quality Care Review, Ohio Academy of Family Physicians; and assistant professor of family medicine, Northeastern Ohio Universities College of Medicine, Akron.

Deborah A. Smith is quality assurance coordinator for ambulatory care services at Medical College of Georgia Hospital and Clinics, Augusta.

Paul M. Spilseth, M.D., M.S., is quality director and staff physician at St. Croix Valley Clinic, Stillwater, Minnesota, and medical director of Lakeview Hospital, Stillwater, Minnesota.

Ruth Srebrenik, M.S., is corporate administrator in the Department of Medicine, St. Luke's–Roosevelt Hospital Center, New York City. She is currently responsible for management of the faculty practice of the Department of Medicine. She was formerly the administrator for ambulatory care at St. Luke's–Roosevelt Hospital. One of her areas of expertise is physician group practice administration, including business development and quality management.

Barbara Toeppen-Sprigg, M.D., is clinical associate director of West Side Family Practice Center, Akron General Medical Center, Ohio; medical director of Quality Care Review, Ohio Academy of Family Physicians; and assistant professor of family medicine, Northeastern Ohio Universities College of Medicine, Akron.

Patricia Warner is associate hospital director and administrator of ambulatory care services at the University of Michigan Hospitals, Ann Arbor.

List of Figures and Tables

Preface

The most natural reaction to a new book on health care quality management is, "Oh no, not another book on quality management! What could possibly be in this book that has not been in 50 others?" This book, however, really is different. Although many other books tell us what we should do, few tell us how to do it. Many other authors tell us why health care quality is so important, but few even attempt to describe the steps for implementing quality assessment programs. This book is different because it is authored by health care professionals who have taken the theory of quality management and transformed it into workable and effective programs. By reading about the authors' experiences, other ambulatory care providers can learn the techniques necessary to develop or enhance their quality management activities.

The term *quality management* is relatively new, and many health care providers still use the term *quality assurance*. In 1990, the Quality Assurance Section of the American Health Information Management Association (formerly the American Medical Record Association) adopted a position statement on quality management in health care. *Quality management* was defined as the "collaborative components and functions enacted by the health care institution to assist it in achieving the goals of delivering high-quality, cost-effective health care services. Components include, but are not necessarily limited to, institution and medical staff monitoring and evaluation activities, utilization management, risk management, infection control and safety." The authors in this publication use both terms: *quality assurance* and *quality management*; they should be considered synonymous. Regardless of which term is used, the process consists of two main activities: quality assessment and quality improvement.

Quality Management in Ambulatory Care describes how various ambulatory health care organizations are defining, measuring, and achieving quality. The book is intended to provide guidelines for quality management in ambulatory care settings, where, until quite recently, the growing quality revolution in health care has gone virtually unnoticed. The text is organized into eight sections. Section one describes three quality management programs from three different perspectives—a private multispecialty clinic, a hospital-based ambulatory care center, and a nursing quality assurance program. The authors present the success factors, as well as the pitfalls to be avoided, in developing a quality management program. Section two describes the challenge of information management and provides direction for the development of a data system to support the ambulatory care quality management program. The authors' experience in designing a computerized data base and information strategy for a hospital-based ambulatory care quality management program provides insights useful in any outpatient setting. Section three details medical record documentation and management issues. Because the ambulatory care medical record serves as the primary data source for quality assessment activities, starting with quality improvement in this area is essential. Not only is excellent record documentation stressed, but a system for improving record storage and confidentiality is outlined.

The assessment and improvement of the clinical quality of ambulatory care services is presented in section four. The foundation of clinical quality review is the development of quality definitions, or standards of practice. Section four begins with an illustration of how one ambulatory care clinic tackled the issue of practice standards formation. Clinical quality assessment applications follow, with detailed, step-by-step descriptions of quality management programs in a multispecialty clinic and a hospital-based ambulatory care program.

Both continuity of care and access are important components of a high-quality outpatient service. Sections five and six describe methods for evaluating the level of quality of these service aspects. The ambulatory care perspective is examined from the payer's viewpoint and in a multidivision outpatient department of a large teaching hospital. Section seven addresses the patient satisfaction survey process, advancing from the basics of questionnaire development to the realities of appraisal and presentation of survey results. Obtaining patient satisfaction data on the quality of ambulatory care services is an important ingredient of quality management. By analyzing patients' reactions to their health care experience, ambulatory care providers can begin to meet and exceed customer expectations. Finally, section eight focuses on the use of practice pattern comparison data to assess the quality of care supplied by individual providers. The authors describe two projects in which aggregate data on "what others are doing" can be used to identify differences that point to ambulatory care quality improvement opportunities.

Quality management in ambulatory care is an evolving science with unique factors not found in the more traditional inpatient programs. The challenges and obstacles described by the authors are real ones. However, common to each author's experience is an enthusiastic confidence that the quality in his or her facility was improved by overcoming these obstacles. As a springboard for the development of new programs and the enhancement of existing ones, this book adds new and time-proven techniques to the growing body of literature on ambulatory care quality management.

Acknowledgments

Health care quality depends in large part on the contributions made by professionals dedicated to the quality management effort. The unsung heroes of ambulatory care quality management—the physicians and quality review practitioners—are the ones who make it happen every day in their facilities. This book could not have been written without these experts, who willingly shared information about what they are doing to improve quality in their organizations. For many, writing about personal achievements does not come easily. Readers should be especially indebted, as I am, to these heroes of ambulatory care quality management who will make our jobs a little easier because they took the time to share.

Section One

Quality Management Program Design

The first step in the ambulatory care quality management process is to design a comprehensive structure that will support the many different functions involved in assessment and improvement activities. The organization must include representation from the various disciplines involved in the ambulatory care system. Leadership must be defined and a program coordinator identified. In this section each author describes the structure and composition of the quality management program that has been successfully implemented in his or her facility. Several program components emerge as common denominators among the programs: definition of purpose, identification of leadership, identification of support staff, standardized reporting, and a well-defined flow of information from the bottom to the top of the organization.

Chapter 1
The Physician Clinic

Paul M. Spilseth, M.D.

Until recently, health care quality assessment and improvement efforts were focused primarily on hospitals. Evaluation of the quality of patient care services began with the patient's entry into the hospital system and ended with discharge. Efforts to measure and improve quality in the outpatient setting were minimal because of the lack of external quality assurance requirements and the diversity of ambulatory care providers. Yet outpatient health care accounts for the largest share of patients' contact with physicians. For example, the average health maintenance organization member makes 4.7 ambulatory care visits each year, whereas fewer than 1 out of 10 members are hospitalized each year.[1] The disparity in quality improvement emphasis has now become apparent, and efforts are already under way in many outpatient settings to develop and implement effective quality management programs. This chapter describes the evolution of a quality management program in a multispecialty physician clinic.

The St. Croix Valley Clinic is a primary care practice made up of 19 physicians. The clinic is located in Stillwater, Minnesota, a suburb of St. Paul, and has more than 55,000 patient visits per year. The clinic maintains all stockholders on the board of directors, and board meetings are held every other month. Five committees with four to five physician members meet each month. The committees are for personnel, operations, administrative, prepaid health care, and quality improvement. An executive committee, composed of committee chairs, meets intermittently for urgent matters that may come up between meetings. The administrator and the clinic president meet with each committee and coordinate communication between committees and the entire staff. All physicians receive an agenda for each committee meeting and are welcome to attend all committee meetings. All physicians are assigned to at least one and possibly two committees so that the governance work is divided among all physicians. Four years ago, with the encouragement of a managed care organization and its own physicians' initiative, the clinic implemented a quality improvement program.

□ Getting Started

Getting started required the formation of a quality improvement committee that was charged with developing and garnering support for a mission statement and making recommendations for an initial investment of financial resources.

The Quality Improvement Committee

The quality improvement committee is composed of a physician chairman, four clinic physicians, a quality improvement coordinator, and two nonphysicians from the clinic staff. The chairman plans meetings, delegates responsibilities, and communicates the activities of the quality improvement program to the rest of the clinic. The quality improvement coordinator is a staff person with enthusiasm, analytical abilities, and medical knowledge and experience—all characteristics important to the success of the program.

The committee meets monthly and functions on an equal basis with the other committees. The quality improvement committee chairman schedules the meetings and prepares and distributes the agenda to all physicians about three days beforehand. Minutes are circulated to the committee members after the meeting, and nonmember physicians receive written reports on special quality improvement projects. At each meeting, the committee receives reports from ongoing projects such as death review, disenrollment, complaints, immunizations, and satisfaction surveys. The nurse supervisor takes responsibility for providing these reports. Special projects are then reported and discussed, and follow-up information on previous projects and proposals for future reviews are presented. The chairman records the minutes of the meeting and sends them to the board of directors. Immediately after the meeting, the chairman prepares the agenda for the next meeting and sets a meeting date. Important issues and project reports are summarized in the monthly clinic newsletter. Figure 1-1 graphically displays the functions of the quality improvement committee.

The Mission Statement

The mission statement clearly defines the purpose, goals, and objectives of the clinic's quality improvement program. This statement, the driving force behind all future quality assessment and improvement activities, includes the following assertions:

The purpose of the St. Croix Valley Quality Improvement Program is to identify opportunities to improve and explore ways to do our work even better than we do it now. We accomplish this purpose by sharing skills, by learning lessons from the past, and by experimenting together.

The goals of the program are the following:

- *Structure:* To evaluate and fix system problems
- *Process:* To understand and improve each step of the work process
- *Outcome:* To measure change in health status related to antecedent care
- *Efficiency:* To obtain improvement in health at the least cost
- *Liability:* To decrease the risk of professional liability
- *Guidelines:* To develop practice indicators that can be used to monitor the uniformity and appropriateness of medical care provided

The objectives of the program are the following:

- To choose two or more aspects of quality to evaluate in depth each year

Figure 1-1. Quality Improvement Committee Functions

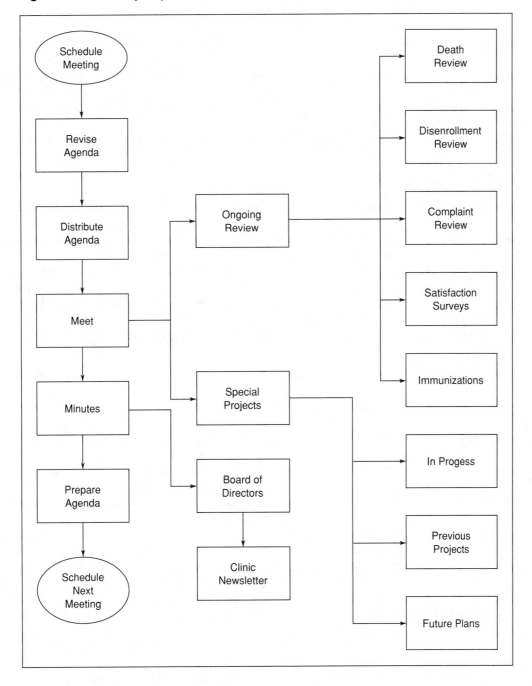

- To include at least 12 medical records per physician per year in these quality studies
- To log all patient and staff complaints and respond to them using various committees depending on the nature of the complaint (the quality improvement committee will receive summaries of all complaints)
- To tabulate and evaluate all deaths and disenrollments for quality-related issues
- To analyze patient satisfaction surveys to identify opportunities to improve

Any project or action of the committee is privileged and not available for malpractice investigation or to anyone outside the organization.

When a draft of the mission statement was completed, the quality improvement committee presented it to the clinic governing board, which includes the medical director and staff physicians. Physicians welcomed the quality improvement ideals, although with some skepticism. Prior experience with hospital quality assurance, which had focused on sanctions, corrective action, and identification of outliers, had not always been positive. The mission statement's positive focus on improvement rather than disciplinary actions was helpful in gaining needed support. The clinic administrator also endorsed the quality improvement initiative. However, the clinic physicians did not simply turn over the quality improvement program to the administrator because the group felt that physician leadership was essential in starting and leading the process.

Financial Resources

The quality improvement initiative also required financial resources. Initial investments included a computer, a laser printer, and word processor and spreadsheet software. Time commitments from physician leaders and nurse supervisors were the major staff resources needed to begin the quality improvement effort. The physician leader of the quality improvement program spends an estimated three hours per month in assessment and improvement activities; the nurse supervisor devotes approximately five hours per month to review and documentation projects. The clinic's budget exceeds $5 million, so this investment was relatively small. One could argue that a much larger portion of the budget should be directed toward achieving high-quality care.

☐ Computerization

Just as a hammer and saw are critical to a carpenter, a computer is essential to quality improvement staff. Although it may be possible to have a quality improvement program in a clinic without using a computer, computerization makes it easier and quicker. It can facilitate the data collection and reporting aspects of quality assessment so that staff can focus on the improvement aspects of quality review. Ongoing monitoring creates more data each month and, along with more data, the need for data organization and storage. Without effective and convenient data storage, it is impossible to compare study results to see whether change occurs.

Whereas for years the computer has had a presence in ambulatory care offices, it has done its work in the back room performing financial functions. The back-room computer dedicated to the finances will usually not serve the quality improvement function because billing staff have first-priority access to this equipment. For most offices, automated medical record applications or computer-generated patient visit reminders are still a prospect for the future. A quality improvement project may be the first opportunity for a clinic physician or nurse to become acquainted with the computer and its data collection and display capabilities.

Therefore it may be necessary to make a financial commitment to purchase a separate desktop computer and laser printer. Because prices for such hardware have dropped to more reasonable levels in recent years, the investment need not be significant. St. Croix Valley Clinic developed a highly sophisticated and effective computerized quality improvement program for less than $3,000 by purchasing an inexpensive Macintosh SE with a hard drive, a GCC Quick Draw™ laser printer, and Microsoft Excel™ spreadsheet and Write Now™ word processing software. Of course, there are alternatives to these choices. Software for a quality improvement program should include a word processor and a spreadsheet. The word processor can be used to produce meeting agendas, meeting minutes, and focused study results. The spreadsheet is simply a series of rows and columns. The data entered into the spreadsheet are easily sorted, alphabetized, or analyzed by any column. High-quality graphs can be generated using the data in the spreadsheet.

☐ Quality Improvement Projects

Assessment and improvement of quality in the clinic setting is divided into two complementary components: ongoing monitoring and special projects directed at a specific problem area. An effective quality improvement program includes both of these elements.

Ongoing Monitors

Ongoing monitors provide regular feedback on important aspects of clinic service. Successful ongoing projects that monitor quality at St. Croix Valley Clinic include complaint review, evaluation of all clinic disenrollments, peer review of all deaths, and patient satisfaction surveys (surveys are described in section seven of this book).

Complaint Review

Although it may be argued that patient complaints have little if anything to do with the quality of medical care provided by the clinic physicians and staff, it is important to remember the two types of quality: quality in fact and quality in perception.[2] *Quality in fact* is that which complies with one's own specifications. It means doing the right thing, doing it right the first time, and doing it on time. *Quality in perception* is more subjective and is based on the customer's experiences. It means delivering the right product that satisfies your customer's needs and expectations of the health care episode. John Pekkanen described the quality-in-perception component of health care delivery when he said, "Being a good doctor . . . has nothing to do with intuition or brilliant diagnoses or even saving lives. It's dealing with a lot of people with chronic diseases that you can't really change or improve. You can help patients. You can make a difference in their lives, but you do that mostly by drudgery, day after day paying attention to details, seeing patient after patient, complaint after complaint, and being responsive on the phone when you don't feel like being responsive."[3] Quality in perception relates to these nonclinical aspects of health care services and is measured by asking the customers whether their needs and expectations have been met. For sustained success, the clinic's quality improvement program must focus on both aspects of quality.

The quality improvement program at St. Croix Valley Clinic measures quality in perception through its ongoing patient complaint review. Providing a formal mechanism for discussion of patient complaints is an important quality improvement process in the clinic, allowing for free exchange of information and setting the stage for professional and personal growth. Patient complaints are recorded and tabulated, and the frequency of specific types of complaints is analyzed for patterns or trends. If a complaint is random, intervention may be tampering, but if a complaint is recurrent, corrective action may be needed. When a complaint is directed to physicians and nurses, the physicians and nurses require confidentiality and sensitivity to allow them to express their side of the story. Such review should be performed with the same standards of judgment that apply to other civil codes of behavior, that is, presumption of acceptable conduct unless proven otherwise. Physicians and clinic staff must feel that their organizations will stand behind them when they make clinical or other patient care judgments in good faith.[4]

One person is designated to receive copies of all complaints. This person may be the clinic administrator or chairman of the quality improvement committee. Sometimes patients are more willing to complain to an administrator because they feel they may need the physician's services in the future and they do not wish to jeopardize their relationship with the physician. Quality improvement leaders must develop an attitude of welcoming complaints, viewing them as treasures and opportunities for targeting improvements. The clinic should make it very easy for patients to document their complaints, supplying suggestion forms and suggestion boxes that are visibly displayed in waiting areas. Patients who ask for their records to be transferred to another clinic are also a potential source of complaints, and suggestions for improvement can be formally solicited during the record transfer process.

Complaint review involves two strategies: immediate action and response and comprehensive evaluation of complaint patterns/trends. The clinic must respond constructively to complaints because it is well known that "of customers who register a complaint, between 54 and 70 percent will do business again with the organization if their complaint is resolved. The figure goes up to a staggering 95 percent if the customer feels that the complaint was resolved quickly."[5]

Immediate Action

When complaints are received, the administrator (or designated coordinator) presents the complaint to the involved person in private and in a sensitive manner. The first step in the complaint investigation is a speedy and thorough investigation of the facts. This should include an interview with all parties involved. Additional input should be solicited from whomever else may have knowledge relevant to the complaint. Direct contact by a peer is preferred to a memo or phone call. If a physician is the person to whom the complaint is directed, it may be better to have another physician relay and investigate the complaint. Of utmost importance is attending to the patient who complained; he or she must receive prompt feedback explaining how the clinic or the attending physician is responding to the criticism. Ideally this reply is given in person or on the telephone. A follow-up letter is a useful way to document the clinic's response, and maintenance of a copy of this letter in the patient's file is helpful if future problems arise. (See figure 1-2 for a diagram of complaint flow at the clinic.)

Analysis of complaints for improvement opportunities occurs at the quality improvement committee level. At committee meetings the administrator summarizes each complaint received, which often stimulates committee discussion of improvement opportunities. Although many complaints may seem unfounded, they can point to persistent quality-in-perception problems that need solving.

After the meeting, the leader records and tabulates the complaints on a computer spreadsheet (see figure 1-3, p. 10), which has columns for documenting the type of complaint, how it was handled, and the improvement possibilities that were identified. Although not shown in the figure, additional space for a brief description of each complaint is also helpful. To maintain their anonymity, physicians and other staff are identified on the complaint summary form with a numbering system. Because this report is computerized, complaints can be sorted by physician/staff and by type of complaint to assist in the identification of patterns that require further investigation.

Evaluation of Trends

The process of receiving, responding to, discussing, tabulating, and analyzing complaints is a long-term project. Over the first few months of the project, the number of complaints may be too small to be significant for trending purposes; however, short-term events can signal customer satisfaction problems. For example, in one month at St. Croix Valley Clinic, three different patients complained that they could not get an appointment with a particular physician. When this information was brought to the physician's attention, he responded by writing a letter to many of his patients explaining why he was less available and suggesting alternative physicians for them to see. As data are gathered and reported over the long term, this ongoing monitoring project will provide trend information that is very useful in demonstrating where the clinic should focus its improvement energies.

Figure 1-2. Process Flow Diagram for Clinic Complaints

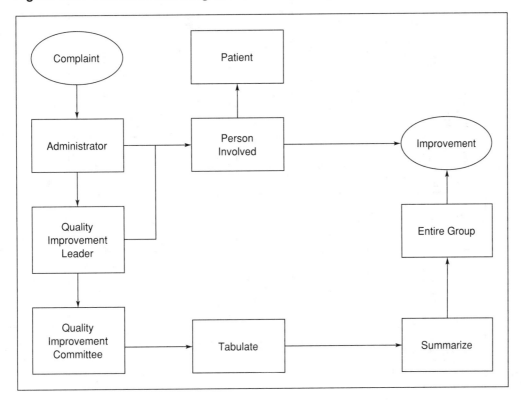

Disenrollment Review

Another ongoing monitoring project that provides feedback about quality is the disenrollment review. When patients leave the clinic to seek health care services elsewhere, a formal mechanism for satisfaction inquiry can be devised. Some patients will ask that their medical records be sent to another clinic or physician. The transfer request form can easily include a question as to why the patient has chosen to leave the clinic. The St. Croix Valley Clinic has used this survey technique to track the reasons for disenrollments for the past four years. At each request for records transfer, the transfer form asks the patient to indicate the reason for the request. The records supervisor collates the answers to this question and summarizes the information for presentation to the quality improvement committee. Over the past four years, the information received from 1,500 disenrolling patients was tracked. Following are the reasons given for requesting transfer of records: moving, 26 percent; insurance change, 50 percent; dissatisfaction, 3 percent; convenience of location, 12 percent; convenience of hours, 0 percent; no reason given, 11 percent. The 3 percent who indicated they were transferring because of dissatisfaction were asked the reason for their dissatisfaction so that the quality improvement committee could follow up on their complaints. The information is also used to assess the clinic's participation in different insurance plans.

Death Review

Death review is one method for evaluating quality in fact. At the completion of the death certificate, the attending physician is asked to complete a death review form. This report asks for a diagnosis, where the death occurred, and whether the patient had a procedure done in the past 7 to 30 days. The physician is also asked to determine whether, in his or her opinion, the death was expected or preventable. The death review form is shown in figure 1-4. St. Croix Valley Clinic asks the attending physician to complete this report because it is felt that in a true quality improvement environment

Figure 1-3. Summary of Patient Complaints

Month	Patient	Physician Number	Type of Complaint					How Responded				
			Systems	Quality Issue	Personality	Communication	Wait (Access)	Referral	Letter	Phone	Personal Communication	Other
Jan.	RH	N/A	X									X
Jan.	ML	8	X							X		
Jan.	JS	N/A	X						X			
Jan.	CN	2	X			X			X	X	X	
Jan.	AH	8	X						X	X	X	
Jan.	SS	N/A					X			X		
Feb.	CN	2	X	X		X			X	X		
Feb.	JS	7		X					X		X	
Feb.	JJ	N/A					X			X		
Feb.	JC	16						X				X
Mar.	JS	16						X		X		
Mar.	ML	N/A					X		X			X
Mar.	DA	N/A					X					X
Mar.	ML	16				X			X			
Mar.	BB	N/A	X						X			
Mar.	LO	N/A	X						X			
Mar.	A	N/A			X					X		
Mar.	LB	15				X				X		

N/A = Not attributed to an individual physician.

Figure 1-4. Death Review Form

Patient Name: _____ Date of Death: _____

Attending Physician: _____

Where Died: _____

Diagnosis: _____

Procedure within past 30 days: _____

Procedure within past 7 days: _____

Check one of the following:

_____ 1. Death was expected for some time.

_____ 2. Although considered possible, death was unexpected at this time.

_____ 3. Death was unexpected.

_____ 4. Other _____

Check one of the following:

_____ A. Death was not reasonably preventable.

_____ B. Death may have been prevented if the patient's correct medical status had been recognized and/or the appropriate therapy given.

_____ C. Death may have resulted from medical intervention with known potential risks.

_____ D. Other

Do the events surrounding this patient's death suggest areas where we can improve future patient care?

_____ Yes   _____ No

Improvement suggestions by reviewing physician:

_____

_____

_____

the physician in attendance at the time of the patient's death is the best person to describe the experience and notice where improvement may have been possible.

The death review form is sent to the quality improvement nurse supervisor, and the data are tabulated on a spreadsheet. One week before the quality improvement committee meeting, the deceased persons' charts are pulled, and the individual cases along with the death review forms are distributed among the physician committee members for review. If the reviewer has comments about a case, he or she will note them on the death review form. At the committee meeting, the reviewer comments on the case and discusses improvement potentials. When the committee completes the review, the death review form goes back to the involved physician with attached comments. A diagram of the complete death review cycle is shown in figure 1-5.

Improvements coming from these efforts are more intangible and more difficult to measure than other quality monitoring activities. However, the following example shows how death review may lead to improvement. A 76-year-old man arrived at the clinic without an appointment and was seen by the emergency physician. Because he was new to the clinic, the man did not have any previous medical records and admitted to rarely seeing health care providers for past problems. He complained about a cough. The physician noted that his chest was clear, but he had an irregular pulse. The physician diagnosed bronchitis and prescribed erythromycin, telling the man to return for further evaluation. One hour later, the man was brought to the hospital after having collapsed at home. During the hospitalization his condition worsened, and he died.

At this point the clinic's death review process began. The reviewer felt that this unfortunate situation could happen to anyone and may have been a random experience.

11

Figure 1-5.   Death Review Process Flow Diagram

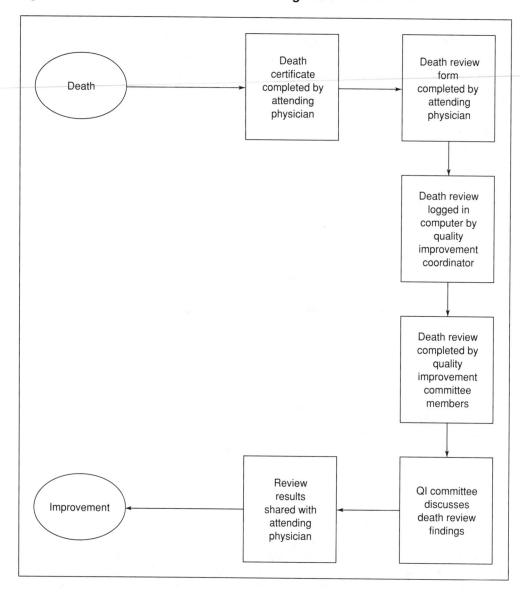

The reviewer did note, however, that the clinical evaluation performed by the emergency physician was rather brief and suggested that a more complete physical examination may have been warranted. As a result of this death review, the quality improvement committee recommended and implemented a policy that states that "all patients new to the clinic who are over age 60 will be given a longer appointment time in order to ensure time for a complete history and physical examination."

Special Projects

Special projects are episodic, in-depth examinations of an area of interest for improvement. The number of potential project possibilities is very large, especially in primary care; the most numerous are diagnosis based. St. Croix Valley Clinic has reviewed its management of patients with hypertension, diabetes, urinary tract infections, colon cancer, estrogen replacement therapy, and *chlamydia* infections. Other topic possibilities include focusing on the management of patients who are referred to another facility for a specific procedure. The clinic has reviewed the appropriateness of tympanostomy tubes, CT (computed tomography) scans of the head, and management of cerebrovascular accidents. The results of diagnostic tests have also been studied, that is, is the clinic responding appropriately to positive tests for *chlamydia*, sexually transmitted disease, and Lyme titers. System problems identified through patient satisfaction surveys or other quality monitoring activities have also triggered special projects. For example, waiting time, after-hours phone calls, or patients' calls to nurses have been evaluated for quality improvement opportunities.

The following steps should be followed in selecting and monitoring special topics for quality improvement: choose a topic, set goals, identify the cases for inclusion, establish review criteria, compile and analyze the data, communicate the results, provide guidelines for improvement, and repeat the process at a later time.

Choice of Topic

The first step in tackling a special quality improvement project is to choose a specific topic for review. Topics may be identified through the ongoing quality measurement process, for example:

- A trend of patient complaints about clinic wait times might prompt a study of office efficiency and patient visit scheduling practices.
- Death reviews might reveal discrepancies in chart documentation, prompting clinic physicians to choose a special project study to evaluate related issues.
- Patients who leave the clinic complain most about the way in which specialty referrals are handled by the clinic's primary care physicians. A discussion of this issue might result in a special project.

Topics for special projects might also originate from the desire to improve overall performance. Opportunities for improvement in all areas of the clinic are limitless, and merely soliciting ideas for improvement recommendations usually results in many topical suggestions for special projects. Ideas for quality improvement projects may also come from the direct patient care experience. Almost any patient can trigger at least one fertile question and possibility for improvement. Reflecting on patients or colleagues who aroused some emotional response in you during the past 48 hours can generate enough questions for a decade of research.

When one starts to think about the various possibilities of study, the list will be long, and it may be difficult to focus the effort effectively. The observations and questions that flood the curious mind must be collected, captured, and evaluated to find the "good ones." The quality improvement committee should choose special project topics by consensus. The committee may select a diagnosis, a procedure, a lab test, or a system issue because of perceived problems, a high variability of practice patterns, a large economic impact, or because clear patient management guidelines in a particular procedure are lacking. Study opportunities that fit naturally with the goals of the majority of clinic physicians and staff are more likely to result in improvements. If the area of study does not have personal meaning, it will become tedious and barren.

Goal Setting

Once the committee chooses a special project topic, the next step is to consider what the project is expected to accomplish. Questions such as the following help to direct and focus the study:

- What is our experience with this problem?
- What guidelines have other groups drawn up?
- What guidelines can we all agree to?
- What will the project cost?

- What necessary function will be achieved by the completion of this task?
- What alternatives exist that can fulfill the same necessary function?
- Does the study do what it is intended to do? Is there a better way of doing it? Is it repetitious? Is it outdated?

Goals should be set as absolute statements prior to the start of the study. An example of goals for the special project of improving patients' adherence to pediatric immunization schedules is:

1. Determine the number of times pediatric patients do not receive their immunizations as required by the clinic guidelines.
2. Identify the cause of variations from the pediatric immunization schedule.
3. Design a method to reduce variations from the pediatric immunization schedule to enhance the quality of preventive patient care given at the clinic.

The special project goals help the quality improvement committee design the study and collect the necessary information to implement the improvement.

Cases for Inclusion

After the committee selects the topic and sets initial goals, the next step is to identify the cases to be included in the review process. The number of cases to be reviewed in the special project must be determined. A rule of thumb is to review all cases if you have only 20 to 30 cases during the study project time frame. If more cases exist, attempt to review at least 10 percent of the study population or 20 cases. If the numerator is too small, the confidence interval for the results gets very large, making measurement imprecise. Reviewing more than 100 cases does not improve precision sufficiently to justify the amount of work necessary to complete these reviews.

The sample population can be any defined group of patients. For example, managed care patients are a defined population, and it is natural to focus on this group for clinical research. The patient sample can come from a number of sources. Using a specific diagnostic code from billing information may be the most accessible and useful data source for names of patients to include in the study. Information from hospital records can help identify cases in which a particular procedure was performed or for whom a specific diagnosis was treated. The hospital can produce a monthly list of births attended by clinic physicians, and the quality improvement committee can use this list to track the immunization status of the children. The laboratory can provide a list of patients with abnormal laboratory values. Managed care companies can provide a list of patients who have had selected procedures. Some lists will be too long; these may be randomly sampled to make the project workable.

Most special projects are by necessity retrospective, but there are drawbacks to this approach. Anyone who has done retrospective review knows that clinic charts do not always have information neatly in one place and that some information may be missing. A preferable method is a concurrent study where information is gathered at the time the procedure is done or at the time the diagnosis is made. Concurrent data collection helps to ensure that the desired information is obtained; however, busy practitioners may not like the additional record keeping or forms to complete.

Review Criteria

Once the committee chooses a topic, sets general goals, and selects the sample of patients, the next step is to establish criteria for the review process. Selecting criteria is an opportunity for creativity. The key quality factors to be included in the study project may be derived from medical literature sources using the literature search capabilities of a hospital medical library. A source of criteria used frequently by physicians at St. Croix Valley Clinic is *A Guide to Clinical Preventive Services: An Assessment of the Effective-*

ness of 169 Interventions.[6] Experts in the clinic may be a source for study criteria, and consultants may be solicited for suggestions.

After the literature has been searched, local experts and specialists have been consulted, and brainstorming has been accomplished, it becomes clear what data to collect. Keep the criteria simple and the number of data items small whenever possible. Complex and numerous review criteria make data collection burdensome and time-consuming. A data collection form should be designed by the quality improvement leader before data collection begins. Figure 1-6 shows a data collection form used for a study of CT scans performed at St. Croix Valley Clinic in 1991.

Data Compilation

When the charts have been reviewed and the review forms completed, the next step is to compile the data. The computer is an essential tool for this work because of its ability to sort and report information in a manner conducive to analysis. Using a spreadsheet program, data elements are entered into the appropriate columns. By sorting and averaging data, one can often see relationships that otherwise would not be perceived. Statistical analysis of averages, ranges, modes, standard deviation, and standard error is usually sufficient. Pie charts, bar graphs, Pareto diagrams, and histograms illustrate data collection results visually and display relationships graphically.[7]

Communication of Guidelines and Results

The next steps in the process are to summarize the study results, analyze the findings, develop guidelines for patient care or quality improvement recommendations, and communicate the results to the entire clinic group. For example, one goal of the special projects that focus on patient management issues is to establish guidelines for how the clinic should deliver high-quality and efficient medical care.[8] Depending on the results of the review process, the study criteria may ultimately become the clinic's patient management guidelines. If the criteria are adopted as the clinic's patient management guidelines at the completion of the study, the criteria are entered into a reference notebook for each physician. New physicians receive a copy of the guidelines derived from all the studies that have been completed to date.

The committee communicates special project results by several methods. When the quality improvement committee has reviewed the outcome and made appropriate comments, it distributes a written summary of the entire project to all physicians. There is also an opportunity to review the study verbally at staff meetings. In addition, the clinic newsletter may summarize the results of the study for the entire staff. Figure

Figure 1-6. CT Scan Study Data Collection Form

Patient Name: _____ Birth Date: _____

Test Date: _____ Performed Where: _____

Diagnosis: _____

Who Ordered Test: _____

Check if: _____ Contrast   _____ MRI also

Reason for Test: _____

Interpretation: _____

Did treatment change as a result of test: _____ Yes   _____ No

Comments: _____

_____

1-7 (on pp. 17–19) shows the completed summary of the head CT scan study at St. Croix Valley Clinic.

Evaluation of Expected Improvements
The final step is to reevaluate the topic to ensure that the expected improvements were realized. A date should be set to look at the improvements made to determine whether the recommendations and guidelines made a difference and whether quality really did improve. For example, the quality improvement committee restudied the use of CT head scans at St. Croix Valley Clinic using the guidelines that came out of the original project. This follow-up study was performed in January 1992, which allowed sufficient time (eight months) for physicians to incorporate the original study guidelines into their practice decisions. This restudy showed a significant decrease in the use of CT head scans for patients complaining of headaches who did not meet the exception criteria. By completing this follow-up study, the quality improvement committee was able to document the effectiveness of their special project in achieving its desired goals.

☐ Strategies for Success

After several years of completing quality improvement projects in the clinic setting, St. Croix Valley Clinic physicians and staff have identified several barriers to success. An awareness of these issues and implementation of the following strategies before starting on a special project can help prevent its failure:

1. *Be prepared for critics:* The first hurdle is to get everyone comfortable with the notion that the quality improvement effort is going to cost them something personally. That is, the time, energy, and other resources that partners, staff, and patients put into studies will not be spent somewhere else. Economists refer to these costs as "opportunity costs." However, in responding to objections it is important to emphasize that the payback will come later and will ultimately save a great deal of time, energy, and resources spent on unnecessary tests, inefficient operations, and so forth.

2. *Enlist support of physicians other than those on the quality improvement committee:* Recognize that the same factors that motivate one colleague may not motivate another. All parties must be convinced that quality improvement adds a new dimension to physician practices, intellectual satisfaction, and excitement of new observations.

3. *Motivate the clinic staff:* The quality improvement leadership must motivate the clinic staff to help in the improvement project. Staff must carry out many of the aspects of the project that do not require a physician's direct involvement. Using available data and devising short and simple protocols can make the data collection process easier. It is important to persuade others that the results of the study could improve care and efficiency. Objections to the project are likely to come from office staff, who may be responsible for contending with increased paperwork or disruptions in patient flow. Counter these feelings by explaining the reason for the study and the expected benefits to patients. Invite staff suggestions on the best ways to incorporate the study into office routine. Communicate the progress of the study often, and graphically if possible.

4. *Be willing to accept something less than a full-blown research project:* Even with a perfect study, there is no assurance of carrying it out. Practice-based research and quality improvement are faced with many obstacles to perfection. The instruments used are subject to validity and reliability problems. For example, the sample may not truly represent the population under study. The nurse may be indisposed or otherwise unavailable at a key point in the study, resulting in

Figure 1-7. Summary of CT Scan Quality Improvement Project

Background

Head CT scans and MRI have simplified the diagnosis of neurologic problems. Some advocate CT scans for all people with dementing illness, whereas others feel that CT scans should be ordered selectively. Computed tomography is useful for diagnosis of subdural hematomas, normal pressure hydrocephalus, brain tumor, and stroke. Other indications include head injury, unexplained focal neurological signs, or inability to reassure the patient without benefit of a CT scan.

Purpose

The purpose of this study was to answer the following questions about head CT scanning at St. Croix Valley Clinic:

1. How many scans do we order for our patients?
2. For what reasons do we order them?
3. How many CT scans are positive? What is the cost per positive test?
4. Who orders them, neurology or primary care physicians?
5. Where are the CT scans performed?
6. Is contrast used?
7. How many patients also get an MRI?
8. What guidelines should we use in ordering CT scans?

References

Simon, D. G. Cost effectiveness of CT and MRI in dementia.
Medical Decision Making 5:335–54, 1985.

Evans, D. A. Prevalence of Alzheimer's disease in a community population of older persons. *JAMA* 262:2551–56, 1989.

Discussion with neurologist, Ken Hoi, M.D.

Study Method

Two insurance plans, GHI and Blue Plus, provided a list of all St. Croix Valley Clinic patients who had undergone head CT scans within the past year. The quality improvement committee retrospectively reviewed clinic charts, collecting the following patient information:

1. Age
2. Date
3. Place where CT scan was performed
4. Diagnosis
5. Reason for test
6. Name of physician ordering CT scan
7. Presence or absence of contrast study
8. Presence or absence of MRI exam performed concomitantly
9. Interpretation of CT scan (cerebral atrophy is considered part of aging and therefore this finding alone was not considered positive)
10. Documentation if patient treatment was changed after the results of the CT scan were known

Study Results

It was reported by GHI and Blue Plus that their patients at the clinic had 62 head CT scans performed during the past two years. With about 10,000 patients enrolled in these two insurance plans, this averages 3 head CT scans per 1,000 patients per year. Seven of the names provided by the insurance plans were excluded from the study (10 percent). In reviewing the clinic charts of these seven patients, five had no record of having had a head CT scan, one had an eye CT scan, and one had an abdominal CT scan. The remaining 55 patients were included in the study.

At an average cost of $300 per head CT scan, the total cost of the 55 exams performed was $16,500. One-fourth of the exams showed a positive interpretation, with the cost per positive test calculated to be $1,179.

In general, CT/MRI costs are rising for patients. Costs per member for all GHI insurance plan patients are shown below. As seen, the costs have increased rather dramatically over the past three years.

GHI cost of CT/MRI per member per month:

1987	$ 0.12
1988	$ 0.19
1989	$ 0.22
1990	$ 0.55

Figure 1-7. (Continued)

Most head CT scans ordered by St. Croix Valley Clinic physicians were done at Lakeview Hospital and at St. Paul Radiology, but a fair number were done at other locations or the location was unknown. This also includes inpatient exams.

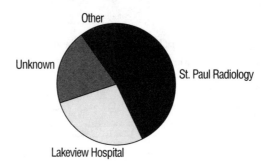

Where Head CT Scans Are Performed

Eighteen patients (33 percent) presented with headache as the reason for the examination. All of these patients had normal head CT scans. The overall results of CT scan interpretations are shown below. NA indicates that no evidence of a CT scan was found in the chart.

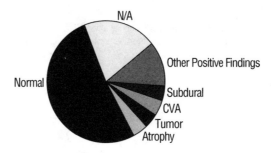

Interpretations of Head CT Scans

The chart below shows who orders head CT scans at St. Croix Valley Clinic.

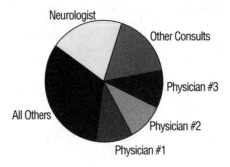

Who Orders Head CT Scans

Figure 1-7. (Continued)

Study Results Analysis

This study helped us to understand our practice as it relates to prepaid patients' utilization and appropriateness of head CT scans ordered by our clinic physicians. Scans are a diagnostic test, and the decision about when to use the test is at the physician's discretion. Sometimes a CT scan is necessary simply to reassure the patient.

Ten percent of the sample was excluded from the head CT scan study, which makes one question the accuracy of billing information being collected by GHI and Blue Plus. Although the insurance plans reported the cost for CT/MRI tests as rising, only 4 (7 percent) of the patients at St. Croix Valley Clinic who had head CT scans also had an MRI performed. Neurologists order most head CT scans. There is some variability in the ordering of head CT scans by physician.

Headache was the major reason given for ordering head CT scans (33 percent), and all of these studies were found to be normal. Findings of all head CT scans showed that approximately 25 percent were abnormal, including tumor, subdural hematoma, CVA (cerebrovascular accident), and other miscellaneous positive findings (such as fluid in the frontal sinus, hydrocephalus, and so forth).

Guidelines

As a result of this study, the following guidelines for ordering head CT scans are recommended.

Head CT scans may be useful for evaluation of:

1. Dementia, especially if the patient is less than 70 years old, the onset of dementia has been recent, and the presentation is atypical
2. Head trauma, where a subdural hematoma is possible
3. Unexplained focal neurological signs or symptoms

Head CT scans are generally not used for:

1. Headache evaluation, unless sudden onset
2. Headache evaluation, unless onset after age 45

---

lost information. Patients may be unwilling to cooperate fully in some aspect of the study. A partner may become impatient with what is deemed "academic nonsense" and refuse to participate any further. Think of the project as a learning experience and recognize that compromises with scientific purity will be needed; however, try not to make so many compromises that the results are meaningless.

☐ Conclusion

"Excellent results are more likely to be achieved when the members of an organization are motivated not by fear of sanctions for inadequate performance, but by pride, accountability, cooperation and loyalty."[9] When quality improvement seeks to promote teamwork among the clinic providers, health care professionals will learn from the past and try new things together. Quality improvement activities teach us how to effectively evaluate what we are doing now and how to do it better in the future.

Using the model described here, it is possible not only to achieve quality in a small-to medium-size medical clinic, but to measure it as well. A mission statement in which the purpose, goals, and objectives are clearly stated is a necessary beginning to the improvement process. The mission statement helps answer the question, "Why should we do quality improvement in our clinic?" Quality improvement projects are both ongoing and episodic. Ongoing projects like death review, disenrollment evaluations, complaint review, and satisfaction surveys provide for measurement of results over time and the identification of improvement opportunities. Special quality improvement projects can be chosen to enhance patient management and strengthen clinic activities. The computer is an essential support tool for the clinic's quality improvement program, helping to store, sort, and present data for effective analysis. Patient management guidelines and more efficient and productive clinic activities are an important outcome of the quality assessment and improvement process.

Quality improvement is a process, not a program. It cannot be completed next month or next year. It should be an integral, ongoing part of the clinic culture. Each project generates data that move physicians and other clinic staff a little closer to their quality goals. The most common question asked about ambulatory care quality review activities is, "Does it make a difference?" The answer is clearly yes!

☐ References

1. Joint Commission on Accreditation of Healthcare Organizations. *Quality Assurance in Managed Care Organizations.* Chicago: JCAHO, 1989, p. 20.

2. Townsend, P. *Commit to Quality.* New York City: Wiley Press, 1987, pp. 5–6.

3. Pekkanen, J. *Doctors Talk about Themselves.* New York City: Delacorte Press, 1988, p. 70.

4. Goldman, H. When patients complain. *HMO Practice* 5(2):51–52, Apr. 1991.

5. Albrecht, K., and Zemke, R. *Service America!* Homewood, IL: Dow-Jones Irwin, 1985, p. 6.

6. U.S. Preventive Services Task Group. *A Guide to Clinical Preventive Services: An Assessment of the Effectiveness of 169 Interventions.* Baltimore: Williams & Wilkins, 1989.

7. Leebov, W., and Ersoz, C. J. *The Health Care Manager's Guide to Continuous Quality Improvement.* Chicago: American Hospital Publishing, 1991.

8. Eddy, D. Guidelines for policy statements: the explicit approach. *JAMA* 263(16):2239–43, Apr. 25, 1990.

9. National Academy of Medicine. *Institute of Medicine Report on Quality of Care in Nursing Homes.* Washington, DC, 1986, p. 188.

Chapter 2

The Hospital-Based Ambulatory Care Department

Emil F. Pascarelli, M.D., and Mary P. Jackson, R.N.

Implementation of an ambulatory care quality assurance program requires the participation of persons who understand the concepts and scope of practice in an outpatient setting. It is also necessary to understand the interdisciplinary nature of ambulatory care. For example, it is not sufficient to assess only the quality of care given by the primary practitioner. The quality assurance program must evaluate all subspecialty care and integrate that into the general assessment program. It is equally important to examine other systems that contribute to the quality of care, such as medical record availability, turnaround time for laboratory and test results, patient waiting time, follow-up of missed appointments, and level of patient satisfaction. Considering these factors, it becomes apparent that quality assurance for ambulatory care involves a broad range of assessments and improvement opportunities. Unless properly organized, an ambulatory care quality assurance program can overwhelm those attempting to implement it, thus compromising the results.

St. Luke's–Roosevelt Hospital Center is a 1,315-bed, voluntary not-for-profit university hospital providing a full range of health care services at two locations. The hospital center includes approximately 40 on-site outpatient clinics providing care in the following areas: primary care medicine (23,000 annual visits), medical subspecialties (19,000 annual visits), general surgery and surgery subspecialties including orthopedics and ENT (34,000 annual visits), obstetrics/gynecology (30,000 annual visits including high-risk prenatal and oncology subspecialties), and a comprehensive pediatric outpatient service (22,000 annual visits). In order to design an ambulatory care quality assurance program to meet the needs of this diverse organization, a dynamic quality assurance structure had to be created (see figure 2-1).

Organizational linkage with the hospital's quality assurance program is provided through the medical staff's ambulatory care committee and the patient services quality assurance committee. Below this interface with the institutionwide structure is the quality assurance program organization for the ambulatory care division. The clinic chiefs ambulatory care quality assurance medical committee oversees the clinical components of quality assessment and improvement. The interdisciplinary ambulatory care quality assurance committee administers the nonphysician aspects of ambulatory care quality review for nursing, administration, social work, and medical records. The

Figure 2-1. Ambulatory Care Quality Assurance Program Organization

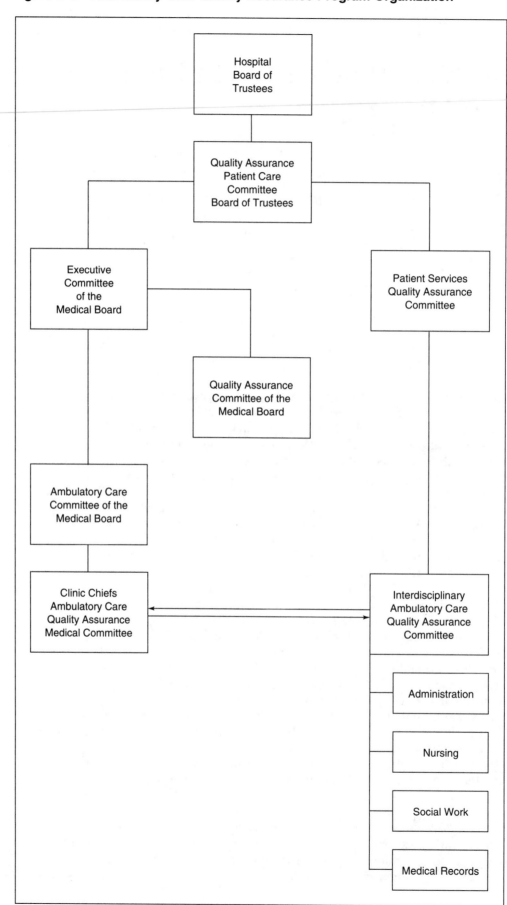

medical director of ambulatory care services sits on both committees to ensure continuity in the quality management process.

☐ Program Development

The crucial steps in the development of a quality assurance program are the following: obtaining high-level support, securing the appropriate leadership and staffing, setting goals and objectives, and defining the program's scope. The manner in which the Ambulatory Care Services Division at St. Luke's–Roosevelt Hospital Center accomplished each of these phases is discussed in the following sections.

High-Level Support

The first step in organizing the ambulatory care quality assurance program is to gain the support and approval of the highest levels of governance in the organization. Tacit approval is insufficient. The ambulatory care quality assurance endeavor not only must be embraced by the governing body, but it must also provide the necessary resources to accomplish the task. The governing body must be made aware of the need for ample resources to support the quality assurance program, which, in ambulatory care, is broad in scope and exceedingly complex. At St. Luke's–Roosevelt Hospital Center, this support was secured by educating the governing body about the importance of quality assessment and improvement. This education was undertaken by the medical director, who met frequently with governing board members to capture their attention and support. Once ambulatory care departments have completed this critical step, development of the program can begin.

Leadership and Staffing

Ambulatory care quality assurance should be organized as a distinct and separate entity even if it is part of the institutionwide quality assurance program. Failure to separate the program in ambulatory care creates the potential for the ambulatory care activities to become obscured and lose identity. Ultimately, the ambulatory care quality assurance program may lose its ability to implement change.

Dynamic leadership is necessary to maintain a high profile for the program. In carrying out his or her activities, the person (or persons) identified with quality assurance can foster a continuing awareness of the existence and need for quality assessment and improvement. The ideal leader is one who has an excellent reputation within the unit and throughout the hospital. He or she must have superior leadership abilities and must also be an excellent communicator and a tireless contributor to the quality effort. Finally, the right choice is someone who has demonstrated the ability to manage complex information-based projects and who has a strong interest in quality improvement and customer satisfaction.[1]

At St. Luke's–Roosevelt Hospital Center, the medical director of ambulatory care is responsible for all quality assessment and improvement activities, ensuring that the following goals and objectives are met:

- Provide a coordinated, comprehensive quality assurance program that involves all departmental activities and operations.
- Provide mechanisms for continuous monitoring of quality in order to identify problems in patient care.
- Establish priorities for problem evaluation and resolution.
- Investigate, review, and assess known or suspected problems, variances, incidents, and complaints.

- Notify the appropriate authorities of pertinent findings.
- Monitor and document that corrective action has been effective in problem resolution.
- Promote improvement in the quality of patient care and services through education, sharing of information, and the development of a commitment to high-quality care.
- Integrate quality assessment findings with staff performance evaluations and with the medical staff reappointment and delineation-of-privileges processes.
- Achieve compliance with the standards set by the Joint Commission on Accreditation of Healthcare Organizations (JCAHO) and with laws and regulations promulgated by the state of New York.

A full-time ambulatory care quality assurance coordinator reports directly to the medical director. She is responsible for the collection, collation, review, analysis, and presentation of the quality assurance findings to the appropriate people and groups. She also is a member of the clinic chiefs committee and the ambulatory care committee of the medical board, providing clerical assistance and collecting/reporting data for their quality assessment and improvement projects.

Physician chiefs from each service are members of the clinic chiefs ambulatory care quality assurance medical committee. This committee identifies areas in which to improve clinical patient care through the use of outcome criteria and selects issues in need of corrective action by the medical staff. The clinic chiefs meet monthly, at least 10 times a year. The committee, in cooperation with physicians working in the various clinics, establishes quality review priorities each year. Figure 2-2 shows the Ambulatory Care Division's clinical quality assurance activities calendar for one year.

The interdisciplinary ambulatory care quality assurance committee monitors and evaluates the nonmedical operational aspects of ambulatory care. The committee uses criteria and indicators of quality derived from performance standards developed by ambulatory administrative/clerical, nursing, and social work staff. Ongoing review is performed by each discipline, and issues that require follow-up are discussed by the committee so that corrective action plans can be developed. Figure 2-3 shows the activities of this committee for one calendar year.

Goals and Objectives

The two major goals of any outpatient quality assurance program are to identify problems or opportunities to improve and then take the steps necessary to achieve the improvements being sought. These goals must be written into the departmental quality assurance plan and communicated to each ambulatory care provider.

As the quality assurance process begins, the goal-oriented assessment and improvement activities should be kept as simple as possible. Do not expect each ambulatory care provider group to schedule more than four quality measurement activities in any one year. As the program evolves, its impact will become greater and its nonthreatening approach will be better appreciated by all participants. When this happens, professional pride and curiosity will be piqued and involvement in multiple assessment and improvement activities will result.

Because no two institutions are alike, it is difficult to predict how the program will unfold. Therefore, a key objective is to keep the structure of the program both simple and flexible so that changes can be made readily. However, it is important to remember that when changes are made—in direction, focus, and so forth—they must tie in to the quality assurance goals originally set in the developmental stages. The questions to be asked are: "Will this quality assurance activity help the organization to better evaluate the quality of patient care provided?" and "Does this scheduled improvement activity have the potential for strengthening the quality of services?" If the answers are yes,

Figure 2-2. Annual Calendar of Clinical Quality Assurance Activities

The following aspects of care are monitored on an ongoing basis in the ambulatory care quality assurance program.

Division	Aspect	Review Schedule
1. All clinics	Problem and medication list	Quarterly
2. All clinics	Admission of outpatient department patients	Monthly
3. Medicine	Management of hypertension	Semiannually
4. Medicine	Management of asthma	Annually
5. Medicine	Management of diabetes	Semiannually
6. Obstetrics/ gynecology	Prenatal care: routine	Quarterly
7. Obstetrics/ gynecology	Prenatal care: follow-up of positive sexually transmitted disease test results	Semiannually
8. Obstetrics/ gynecology	Prenatal care: follow-up of positive HBsAG (hepatitis B surface antigen) test results	Semiannually
9. Obstetrics/ gynecology	Prenatal care: follow-up of negative Anti-D titer results	Semiannually
10. Obstetrics/ gynecology	Prenatal care: follow-up of rubella titers below 1:8	Semiannually
11. Obstetrics/ gynecology	Routine gynecological check-up	Quarterly
12. Pediatrics	Management of asthma	Quarterly
13. Pediatrics	Management of patients with elevated blood lead levels	Annually
14. Pediatrics	Health supervision/prevention	Quarterly
15. Pediatrics	Management of patients with otitis media	Annually

Note: Ad hoc studies are generated based on monthly review of quality assessment data sources.

Figure 2-3. Annual Calendar of Interdisciplinary Quality Assurance Activities

The following quality indicator data are collected on an ongoing basis in the ambulatory care quality assurance program.

Department	Quality Indicator	Review Schedule
1. Clinic administration	Patient access/appointment	Monthly
2. Clinic administration	Patient no-show rates	Monthly
3. Clinic administration	Clerical assignment completion	Monthly
4. Clinic administration	Patient no-show follow-up	Monthly
5. Medical records	Chart retrieval rates	Monthly
6. Nursing	Patient education and/or chart documentation	Monthly
7. Social work	Referral documentation	Monthly
8. Medicine (TRACS*)	Continuity	Monthly
9. Medicine (TRACS*)	Patient access	Monthly
10. Medicine (TRACS*)	No-show rates	Monthly

*TRACS is an acronym for Teaching Residents Ambulatory Care Skills, a primary care teaching program within the Department of Medicine of St. Luke's–Roosevelt Hospital Center.

then the quality assurance endeavor should be undertaken. If the answers are no or "not sure," then rethink the objectives because they may not be in keeping with the quality assurance program goals.

In addition to overall quality assurance program goals, the ambulatory care department may wish to establish more specific objectives that are also documented in the quality assurance plan. Following are some examples of objectives that also serve as a road map to ensure proper focus of the ambulatory care quality assessment and improvement process:

- Health care services are appropriate to the needs of the patient and are of acceptable medical quality based on current medical knowledge.
- Delivery of health care services is provided in an efficient manner with a reduction in unnecessary or avoidable delays in services.
- There is improvement where suboptimal elements of care or service are identified.
- There is a mechanism to coordinate the findings of quality assessment and improvement activities with continued medical and staff education.
- The results of quality assessment and improvement activities are communicated to the administrative leadership and each ambulatory care provider.

Scope

The scope of the program should be comprehensive, requiring the study of all the elements necessary to produce the desired results. As already noted, ambulatory care quality assurance inherently has a broad scope that assesses the efforts of many interacting disciplines. These disciplines might include administration, nursing, social work, medical records, episodic and continuing care, and systems monitoring. Because of the involvement of so many disciplines, it becomes necessary to delegate responsibility to key persons who report to a central committee that documents and integrates quality assurance results, such as the interdisciplinary ambulatory care quality assurance committee at St. Luke's–Roosevelt Hospital Center.

In some cases, outcome-oriented, disease-specific studies will require cooperation of several disciplines, including those not traditionally seen as ambulatory care providers. Such studies are often sparked by an isolated finding. For example, St. Luke's–Roosevelt Hospital Center found that asthmatic patients who frequently use the hospital emergency services often do not receive their primary care there but simply work in the neighborhood. Further study showed that many of the patients have a significant psychiatric illness or substance abuse problem that complicates compliance with their medical regimen for asthma. Analysis of patient records and interactions with emergency staff showed that many patients lacked education about their illness and there was a need to evaluate the patients' home conditions. Clinic physicians felt that more frequent primary care visits would enable the patients' asthma to be better controlled, thereby preventing the need for emergency care. Ultimately, the quality assurance committee recommended the development of an organized asthma care program to address these identified concerns. Although these discoveries had nothing to do with the original objective of the emergency services asthma care study, they ultimately benefited the patient population in a number of ways.

☐ Program Priorities

In that many ambulatory events will occur that signal the need for quality improvement activities, it is critical to establish priorities. There are never enough people and never enough time available to work on every quality improvement project, so these resources must be prioritized for maximum effectiveness in quality improvement. The ambulatory care quality assurance plan of St. Luke's–Roosevelt Hospital Center recommends that departments consider the following issues when they select quality improvement projects:

- Patient outcomes (risk or presence of mortality/morbidity)
- Frequency of occurrences or complaints and duration
- Problems that cross departmental lines
- Financial impact
- Liability concerns

Using these criteria, ambulatory care providers select quality assessment and improvement projects that will result in the biggest gain. For example, the following questions can be asked: "If I measure this attribute of patient services and ultimately make improvements in the process of health care delivery, will I significantly improve patient outcomes? Will I significantly improve patient satisfaction? Cross-departmental cooperation?" By truthfully answering such questions, ambulatory care providers have found the focus of their improvement activities to be on the 20 percent of systems that create 80 percent of the quality concerns. Unlike the institution that has merely a paper program, St. Luke's–Roosevelt Hospital Center's quality assurance program has produced measurable and significant quality gains. Each of these areas of concern is discussed in the following sections.

Patient Outcomes

One of the most important signal events is an untoward incident involving a patient. Much can be learned from investigating an encounter in which errors have led to a less-than-satisfactory patient outcome. Because of the adverse outcome, these incidents receive the highest priority for analysis. These are typically the type of cases that warrant an in-depth review of care with respect to all the disciplines. In addition, they are excellent for teaching and generally elicit a great deal of interest, especially on the part of the providers directly involved in the care. For example, in reviewing one type of event, *hospital admission for adverse results of outpatient management*, several different aspects of ambulatory care can be discussed:

- Was the patient's diagnosis delayed? Could earlier diagnosis in the outpatient clinic have prevented the admission?
- Was the admission attributed to drug therapy initiated while the patient was an outpatient, that is, bleeding while on anticoagulants; gastrointestinal bleeding while on aspirin, Butazolidin, or Indocin; hypokalemia (potassium level below 3.0) while on diuretics or digoxin; digitalis toxicity; other serious drug reactions? Could outpatient management have been changed to prevent this hospitalization? Was patient education adequate?
- Was the admission due to a complication following outpatient care, that is, malunion/nonunion of fracture; irradiation burns; wound infections; bleeding following termination of pregnancy? Is there a pattern of complications that requires further investigation?
- Was the admission for a disease for which immunization is available, that is, measles, mumps, polio, diphtheria, or tetanus? Could the outpatient department have effected an improvement in the patient's immunization status?
- Was the admission caused by the patient's failure to respond promptly to recommended treatment, that is, the patient did not follow up with diagnostic tests ordered by the physician? Could the clinic have improved the continuity of care?

- Was the admission caused by a delay in necessary treatment? For example, was the patient unable to get an appointment at the clinic? Was the outpatient diagnosis in error and treatment delayed because of this error?

The exploration of any of these issues could result in the improvement of a process that would have a favorable impact on the delivery of care.

Frequency of Occurrence and High Risk

Another high-priority reason for performing quality assurance activities in a given area is that the category of care involves a large number of patients at risk. For example, studies on a group of patients with specific diagnoses such as diabetes or hypertension might be performed because of the high risk that inappropriate management will compromise the quality of patient care. Studies involving large numbers of patients at high risk make up one of the more prominent categories of quality assurance and usually afford a considerable degree of opportunity for change. This quality review category also lends itself to ongoing follow-up reviews to determine whether patient management changes that have been implemented have had an impact on the quality of care.

This outcome-oriented, high-volume, high-risk approach to quality review is the quintessential element of the quality assurance program. In evaluating the quality of care provided to individual patients with specific diagnoses, there is the potential for a broad in-depth investigation. Experience has shown, though, that the review process should begin simply with the inclusion of a few basic patient management criteria. For example, the primary care clinic at St. Luke's–Roosevelt Hospital Center regularly evaluates the quality of care provided to patients with hypertension. Charts of patients with a diastolic pressure of 110 or greater are evaluated using the following 11 criteria:

1. Blood pressure was taken and documented on each clinic visit.
2. The appropriate antihypertensive medication was ordered.
3. Chart documentation included the patient's level of compliance with medication ordered.
4. An appropriate time was set for a follow-up visit.
5. The patient's weight was monitored.
6. The appropriate diet was ordered for the patient.
7. Chart documentation included the patient's level of compliance with the diet ordered.
8. The patient was referred to a dietitian for dietary counseling.
9. Blood pressure improved with medical regimen.
10. The patient kept scheduled clinic appointments.
11. Determination was made of evidence that the patient has a history of psychiatric problems and/or substance abuse that would affect clinical course and patient compliance.

Over time the criteria may be expanded and thereby the scope of review of care may be broadened for that particular group of patients.

Cross-Departmental Problems

Problems that cross departmental lines often signal system problems that represent a breakdown in communication or process failures. Some pioneers of quality improvement claim that process problems (not people or their performance) are responsible for 80 to 90 percent of the quality problems that plague health care organizations.[2] For this reason, cross-departmental issues should receive high-priority attention from the ambulatory care quality assurance program.

When opportunities for improvements are identified by other departments, the ambulatory care services unit must be willing to support multidepartmental process improvement projects. This support might be as simple as appointing an ambulatory care service representative to a quality improvement team, such as one formed by the hospital to improve the process of surgery scheduling. Alternatively, the ambulatory care services department might sponsor a quality improvement team to investigate ways of enhancing communication among the diagnostic departments and the ambulatory clinics.

Financial Impact

The cost of poor quality can significantly influence an ambulatory care department. Whereas the clinical components of health care may receive higher priority for improvement activities, the ambulatory care department may choose to also look at the financial aspects of its performance. In choosing their quality assessment and improvement projects, ambulatory care providers should be encouraged to consider the financial savings that will be gained by making improvements. Quality problems usually cost the institution money in terms of rework, extra paperwork, duplication of staff efforts, non–value-added activities, and so forth. Examples of quality indicators that measure issues of financial importance, as well as clinical relevance, for ambulatory care providers include the number of:

- Mislabeled/misplaced specimens
- Misplaced/misfiled/misidentified laboratory or radiographic findings
- Rejects/repeats of X-ray examinations
- Surgeries canceled because of new findings not detected by the primary care physician during preoperative evaluation
- Client records missing/unavailable at the time of scheduled appointment

Liability Concerns

Although liability control is not the highest-priority reason for performing quality assessment and improvement activities, it is usually inherent in many quality assessment and improvement projects. Recognizing the potential for discovering risk management concerns in the clinically focused quality assurance activities of ambulatory care providers is important. Liability control, then, becomes another reason for selecting particular assessment or improvement ventures. For example, the following quality indicators measure the quality of clinical services as well as provide information essential to the ambulatory care provider's liability control activities:

- Injury to clients, visitors, or staff
- Venipuncture complications (hemolyzed specimens, hematoma, infection, and so forth)
- Failure to verify laboratory results that fall outside established quality control limits
- Radiologic studies performed on pregnant women
- Physician orders for therapy/medications that exceed recommended frequency or dose

Other Priority Considerations

In the delivery of hospital-based ambulatory care, numerous *regulatory agencies* periodically assess the various components of ambulatory care services. For example, the Joint

Commission on Accreditation of Healthcare Organizations (JCAHO) has established standards that are used in periodic surveys of member institutions for the purpose of accreditation. In addition, numerous states have strict criteria that are often superimposed on those of the JCAHO. If in the process of a JCAHO survey problems are discovered, this may result in a type I recommendation. "A type I recommendation is a recommendation or group of recommendations that should receive the highest priority in the hospital's plans for improvement. The hospital's progress will be monitored by the Joint Commission through focused surveys or written progress reports at stated times during the accreditation cycle."[3] Once a type I recommendation has been given, a specific time frame may be imposed on the provider of care to make corrections as expeditiously as possible. The ambulatory care quality assurance process would place type I recommendations at high priority for improvement.

Other areas ripe for the identification of quality improvement opportunities are *new programs or procedures.* When procedural changes occur in an ambulatory care setting, these need to be evaluated as an element of the delivery of care so that a determination can be made about their efficacy. For example, new registration procedures for patients might have a significant impact on waiting time and ultimately on the time it takes to see the provider.

Staffing changes have the potential to produce dramatic dislocations in the provision of care. This is especially true if staff reductions are initiated for the purpose of economy. In the latter circumstances the potential for adverse outcome increases. Quality assurance staff must therefore be alert and monitor the areas where staff reductions occurred until stability returns to the system.

Although computerized information systems may ultimately improve the flow of information to the provider, during the transitional phase of their installation and implementation difficulties may arise that warrant quality monitoring. The *creation of any new programs or services* can pose unique difficulties for individuals or groups of providers. Generally, these programs require new staffing and new systems to function adequately. For example, the creation of a comprehensive breast screening program may require the integration of several different services. To provide the maximum efficiency of care for patients in this setting, the examining physician must have (preferably at the time of the first visit) the capability of doing mammography and performing needle aspiration biopsy. Such a program, then, requires coordination with radiology, surgery, and pathology services to provide optimal patient care.

Although often ignored, the *efficacy of established health care service programs* must be periodically assessed. Such an assessment may result in beneficial changes to the program, uncover inefficiencies, or even indicate that a program is no longer providing a useful service and should be terminated. Programs with major teaching potential need frequent critical review. Obviously students, residents, and others depend on a good-quality educational experience in order to advance themselves professionally. It is incumbent upon the quality assurance program to ensure an environment where education can prosper.

Providing good ambulatory health care requires an *investment in equipment and other assets* needed in today's technologically oriented environment. An efficient quality assurance process can do much to protect these assets. Quality control is often separated from the more clinically oriented quality assurance; however, it is the belief at St. Luke's–Roosevelt Hospital Center that quality control should be closely linked and preferably integrated with a comprehensive quality assurance program. It is critical to ensure that equipment used in patient care procedures is not obsolete and inappropriate when compared to community standards. It therefore becomes necessary to make recommendations to the providers of services to invest in new equipment as needed to continue to maintain high standards of care.

Finally, the quality assurance program must address those *areas of particular interest expressed by the providers of care.* In addition to having potential for significant educational impact, highlighting these areas will nurture interest, cooperation, and support of the quality assurance effort. Such interest might involve the physician's concerns about the impact of the care provided in the outpatient setting and its relationship to the hospital admission. In this case the key question is, "Could admission to the hospital have been prevented by providing more effective outpatient care?" Initial quality review activities should focus on those areas where the least amount of resistance will be encountered. Interested, enthusiastic, and cooperative physicians will make the task easier.

The establishment of priorities is a critical component of the quality assurance process. Creating these priorities can serve to clarify the goals of the quality assurance effort. However, setting the priorities is more of an art than a science because it depends on a variety of factors that may vary from institution to institution and change at any given time. The recognition of the dynamic aspect of this process can help to ensure success of the quality assurance program.

☐ Quality Assurance Methodology

Methodology is the body of methods, rules, and postulates employed by the quality assurance program, including specific procedures, that will enable the program staff to carry out its goals. The procedures described here include identifying indicators, setting expected levels of performance, collecting the data, developing reports and disseminating information, and implementing changes.

Identification of Indicators

One of the most common methods for measuring quality in ambulatory care is the use of indicators, or benchmarks. Indicators are generally events or specific circumstances that trigger a quality assurance review. For example, a blood sugar level consistently above 300 milligrams per deciliter (mg/dl) in a diabetic patient under treatment is an indicator of the quality of care provided to that patient. Another indicator could be hypertensives under treatment whose diastolic blood pressure remains greater than 110 millimeters mercury (mm Hg).

The presence of these events, as measured by indicators of quality, prompts action by the quality assurance committee. This action usually leads to the creation of criteria for an in-depth evaluation of the process of patient management. For example, in the case of the diabetic whose blood sugar is found to be elevated, criteria can be used to measure and evaluate the appropriateness of the various facets of care, which might include medication, diet, and patient compliance.

In general, ambulatory care providers can choose from two types of quality indicators: sentinel event and rate-based indicators. *Sentinel event* indicators measure the occurrence of a "serious" event, for example, patient admission to the hospital within 24 hours following a clinic visit. *Rate-based* indicators measure the frequency of an event that is expected to occur occasionally, for example, X-ray repeat or reject. The primary difference in use of these two types of indicators is in the analysis of results. One hundred percent of all events that are identified with sentinel event indicators require additional peer review to assess the quality of care provided. Quality assessment activities for rate-based indicators, on the other hand, do not begin until the reported results trigger a predetermined threshold, that is, a percentage of occurrences within a particular time frame. For X-ray repeats or rejects, this threshold might be set at 5 percent, and further action is taken only when the reported rate exceeds 5 percent. Thresholds are discussed further in the following section.

Expected Performance Levels

Prior to beginning data collection for quality indicator measurements, each ambulatory care provider group must set quality expectations, or thresholds for evaluation. Thresholds for sentinel event indicators of quality are always set at 0 percent, because these indicators identify serious events that require action (peer assessment) every time they occur. Rate-based indicator thresholds may be set at something other than 0 percent because these indicators measure events that are expected to occur periodically.

Thresholds for rate-based indicators should be established with input from the ambulatory care provider groups whose quality is being measured by the indicator. For example, a primary care clinic may wish to measure the quality of its patient care, using as an indicator the number of patients with known malignancy whose record lacks temperature and weight documentation for every clinic visit. In this case, both the physicians and clinic staff should agree on an acceptable level of compliance. Because circumstances outside the physicians' or clinic staff's control may cause this documentation to be missing, an acceptable standard might be 90 percent or even less. This level of acceptable quality must be a joint decision by all involved providers.

Thresholds for evaluation can also be derived from current medical literature. For example, ambulatory care providers might establish 100 percent as their threshold for compliance with the practice parameters developed and published by medical professional societies. For a listing of guidelines and practice parameters developed by these societies, contact the particular societies or the American Medical Association in Chicago.

Data Collection

Because indicators of quality can be derived from a variety of data sources, no stone should be left unturned in examining data for applicability to the ambulatory care program. Creative and interested staff can identify events requiring more in-depth review from laboratory logs showing abnormal findings, admission listings, medical records, policy manuals, and a variety of other material. If data sources such as these are not readily available, they should be developed in order to capture information to be used in the evaluation process.

Report Development and Information Dissemination

Reporting of results can begin once the quality assurance process is completed, that is, once the data are collected and examined. Reports of findings will proceed in two directions. The first direction involves the transmission of reports to appropriate committees at various levels of governance within an institution. This information provides administrators with data relating to the quality of care, thereby allowing them to take necessary remedial action. When quality assurance findings uncover a problem that cannot be solved by the ambulatory care division alone, communication of results to the highest levels of governance is helpful in obtaining the necessary support and funding. The second path along which this information travels leads to individual providers directly concerned with the care of patients. Quality assurance reports provide feedback on their individual practices and ultimately result in changes in their approach to patient care.

Because quality assurance data are disseminated so widely and theoretically are available to outside regulatory agencies, every effort must be made to safeguard confidentiality of the patient and provider, thereby maintaining the integrity of the quality assurance program. The quality assurance program should have a confidentiality statement that describes what data are protected from release to outside groups and how this information is secured to prevent unauthorized release. The quality assurance confidentiality policy for St. Luke's–Roosevelt Hospital Center is shown in figure 2-4.

Implementation of Changes

When quality indicator data reveal an unacceptable variation from preestablished thresholds or when case review uncovers a practice pattern requiring change, the improvement phase of the quality assurance program is set in motion.

Taking corrective action when a problem is identified is usually not a simple matter and may require changing long-established work habits or making substantial changes in clinical or administrative policies and procedures. In general, the following four quality improvement steps should be taken:

1. *Analyze the situation.* This may require the collection of additional information to identify the problem that is evidenced by the quality indicator data. For example, without performing an in-depth analysis of the reason for multiple repeat emergency visits for asthmatic patients, St. Luke's–Roosevelt Hospital Center would probably have overlooked the problems of patient education and home care conditions. In analyzing the situation, care must be taken to include the physicians and clinic staff involved in providing the services. This may require the

Figure 2-4. Policy on Confidentiality

Subject: Confidentiality of Quality Assurance/Risk Management Data

Policy Statement: The following policy has been adopted in order to ensure the confidentiality of all data collected for the quality assurance/risk management programs.

1. All proceedings, documentation, records, or committee action related to the performance of medical review; participation in a program carried out as required by state law; incident reporting or investigation for renewing professional privileges and association, including information submitted, collected, or prepared for the purpose of evaluating and improving patient care; reducing morbidity and mortality; and determining that health care services are professionally indicated or performed in compliance with applicable standards, shall be kept confidential. Such information shall not be disclosed to anyone pursuant to a request as noted in paragraph 2, without the express permission of the vice-president for legal affairs and the vice-president for professional affairs. All hospital quality assurance activities are presumed to be governed by this provision.

2. Notwithstanding the above, if the Hospital receives a request for information from another medical care facility regarding a practitioner who has applied for privileges, the Hospital shall provide information regarding (i) pending malpractice actions or misconduct proceedings, (ii) judgments or settlements of malpractice actions or any findings of professional misconduct, and (iii) any incident of professional misconduct required by law to be reported to the Department of Health.

3. Whenever possible, minutes, records, and all other quality assurance material and information should be labeled "quality assurance committee information compiled in accordance with statute and regulation."

4. Once a determination is made that a person or entity outside the Hospital is legally entitled to access to quality assurance information, the person(s) subject to investigation should be notified.

5. Statements made by any person in attendance at a quality assurance committee meeting who is a party to an action or proceeding regarding the subject reviewed are subject to disclosure. Therefore, it is advisable that quotes and statements by persons in attendance at such meeting or proceedings not be included in minutes.

6. Internal access to the quality assurance records and information noted in paragraph 1, including physician profiles, are strictly controlled. Knowledge of these files and access to them are afforded only to those in the Hospital who need to refer to such information. Reasonable access for committee or departmental members must be maintained to facilitate appropriate decision making based on information contained in the minutes. The medical board should develop mechanisms for determining the individuals who will retain the records and the procedure for allowing access to them and forward their recommendations to the patient care committee of the board of trustees, which may either establish rules governing access or delegate to an individual or individuals the right to make the determination.

---

formation of a quality improvement team charged with examining the health care process identified as a problem area. The analysis may take the most time of any quality improvement phase, but it is the step most critical to project success.

2. *Identify the causes of problems.* It is an accepted fact that 80 to 90 percent or more of problems have a root cause that is due to the failure of a health care system or process and not to the failure of an individual provider. This knowledge must be kept at the forefront of discussion of problem causes—the goal is to improve the process, not to look for a scapegoat. This attitude will greatly enhance the ability to identify and solve problem areas.

3. *Decide whether available data are sufficient and usable to determine causes.* Once the causes of unacceptable quality variations are hypothesized, it may be necessary to gather additional information to substantiate the root cause of the problem. In the case of the asthmatic patients returning frequently to the emergency department, it was necessary to collect data to validate that patient education and home conditions were the contributing factors to this quality concern.

4. *Determine the best course of action.* This step is simplified if the homework on root cause identification has been performed well. For example, once it became clear that multiple emergency visits for asthmatic patients were caused by problems related to patient education and home conditions, the action—development of an asthma care program—became the most logical endeavor. Furthermore, because the quality improvement project included all involved disciplines in the process of analysis and root cause identification, the long-term changes required by this action were more readily accepted by all physicians, clinic, and hospital staff.

After implementing action plans, time must be allotted to allow the changes to mature and take hold. At the end of the maturing process, the changes can be monitored and reevaluated to determine whether they have produced a positive result. If the desired result has not been achieved, regroup and start the process again. This cyclic approach to quality improvement exemplifies the basic tenet of ambulatory care quality assurance: The job is never finished—there is always something new to evaluate and always something old to reassess.

□ Conclusion

The following guidelines may be helpful in organizing and carrying out quality assurance goals:

- Start simply, with a commonsense approach. Focus on tangible solutions to tangible problems.
- Keep the quality assurance program flexible.
- To get maximum benefit from efforts, leave no stone unturned in examining the applicability of all existing activities in the institution that can be tied to the quality assurance program.
- Start the ambulatory care process where the least resistance is encountered, that is, with the most cooperative groups of physicians and administrators.

Ambulatory care quality assurance is a multifactorial evaluation of a multidisciplinary activity. Evaluation is often frustrating and complex, yet success is best achieved by a simple straightforward approach. Despite the numerous obstacles, the process has great potential for producing meaningful change and improving the quality of patient care.

☐ References

1. Berry, T. *Managing the Total Quality Transformation.* New York City: McGraw-Hill, 1991, p. 18.

2. Leebov, W. *The Quality Quest: A Briefing for Health Care Professionals.* Chicago: American Hospital Publishing, 1991, pp. 14–15.

3. Joint Commission on Accreditation of Healthcare Organizations. *Accreditation Manual for Hospitals.* Chicago: JCAHO, 1992, p. xxvii.

Chapter 3

The Nursing Quality Assurance Program in Hospital Ambulatory Care Services

Deborah A. Smith

The Ambulatory Care Service Department of the Medical College of Georgia provides quality patient care through 17 clinics with 88 subspecialties. The department serves patients from various areas of the state as well as from other states in the Southeast. Although the hospital has been accredited by the Joint Commission on Accreditation of Healthcare Organizations for many years, the Ambulatory Care Service Department has been included in the accreditation process only since 1987. Because the accreditation process looks at the quality of care provided, the department developed its own definition of quality: care that is "effective in bettering the health status and satisfaction of a population, within the resources that society and individuals have chosen to spend for that care."[1]

This chapter describes the development and implementation of a hospital-sponsored ambulatory care quality assurance (QA) program for nursing staff. Administrative support, development of the QA plan, and the monitoring and evaluation process are discussed. In particular, the selection of aspects of care, indicators/criteria development, data collection, evaluation, and reporting are highlighted.

☐ Support of Program Development

The success of the QA program in the Ambulatory Care Service Department at the Medical College of Georgia is due in part to commitment from hospital administration; the ambulatory services director, the ambulatory care management team (ACMT), which is composed of nurse managers from each clinic; and the medical staff ambulatory care committee, which is composed of physicians practicing in the ambulatory clinics. In support of the institution's mission to provide quality care and service excellence, these individuals and groups established the quality assurance program in the ambulatory care services area. The program's success is also a result of internal desire to positively influence the caring aspect of patient management through everyone's involvement in quality assessment and improvement. The shared responsibility of both administrative and clinical staff is vital to the existence of a progressive quality assurance program.[2]

Numerous efforts were made to solidify commitment to an ongoing QA program. A full-time quality assurance coordinator position was created to facilitate development and coordination of the QA program and to serve as a focal point for accreditation issues and requirements. Additional educational funds were allotted to the Ambulatory Care Service Department to ensure access to current knowledge of QA issues and trends. Initially the ACMT met frequently with the QA coordinator to design the QA plan. The clinic staff met with the coordinator to develop specific monitors for their clinics. Although the QA concept had been relatively vague in the department, the assistant hospital director, the director of ambulatory care services, the clinic managers, and staff were cooperative and patient as QA program development and implementation got under way.

☐ Quality Assurance Plan

The QA plan serves as a road map for assessing the quality of patient care and staff competency. The plan outlines the philosophy, purpose, goals, scope, and organization and responsibilities of the QA program. To successfully monitor patient care and support staff performance, well-structured and consistent guidelines are necessary, and the components of the plan should be clearly defined.

Philosophy

The philosophy is a concise yet clear description of beliefs and concepts of the organization's perception of quality care. The philosophy of the QA program in the Medical College of Georgia's Ambulatory Care Service Department reflects the ideology of the entire institution.

Health care professionals are accountable for providing optimal, high-quality patient care in a safe, cost-efficient, and therapeutic manner. A well-developed QA program is an efficient mechanism for evaluating and monitoring the quality of care provided, and for instituting appropriate plans to improve the quality of care.

Purpose

The purpose describes what the facility intends to achieve by having a QA program. For the Ambulatory Care Service Department of the Medical College of Georgia, the purpose of the QA program is described as follows:

> To provide an ongoing process that will promote excellence in health care delivery. This process systematically monitors and evaluates the quality, appropriateness, and cost of care based on current standards of patient care, standards of practice, policies, procedures, and protocols. The program will provide direction for needed changes, which will result in improved quality of care and efficient use of resources.

Goals

The goals of the QA program, which should be clearly defined in the QA plan, identify the expected outcome of the program in very objective statements. Some goals of the QA program at the Medical College of Georgia are the following:

- To identify opportunities to improve care based on a wide variety of data sources including, but not limited to, current monitoring, checklists, incident reports, patient surveys, staff concerns, current practices described in the literature, infection control, and utilization review reports

- To validate for the consumer that high-quality patient care is rendered
- To recommend corrective action to the appropriate persons for problems identified
- To follow up and document that corrective action was taken and the desired results were obtained
- To demonstrate the appropriateness of patient care services provided to each patient
- To reduce the number of potential unusual occurrences related to health care services
- To communicate ambulatory care service QA activities to the hospital QA committee (which includes physicians)
- To promote the concept of peer review and QA among nursing, clerical and administrative personnel, and physicians in the Ambulatory Care Service Department
- To improve the level of patient satisfaction

Scope

The scope of the QA program lists the range of activities and methodologies that will be used to monitor and evaluate patient care and services. The scope of the QA program at the Medical College of Georgia encompasses the involvement of 17 clinics and addresses the following:

- Professional status qualification (credentialing):
  —Verification of licensure
  —Continuing education
  —Orientation (including competency assessment) and certification
  —Performance appraisal
- Risk management:
  —Incident reporting
  —Unusual occurrence trending
  —Quality control rounds
  —Review of number of error reports
  —ACMT financial chart audit
  —Safety committee representation
- Standards:
  —Staff development standards
  —Patient education standards
  —Performance standards
  —Standards of care
  —Standards of practice
  —Policies and procedures
- Monitoring and evaluation activities
- Patient care studies
- Relationship with quality assurance activities of other departments/services
- Participation in hospital QA program
- QA plan evaluation

Organization and Responsibilities

According to Richards and Rathbun, large health care providers should clearly define the QA responsibilities of participants and should include all levels of the organization.[3] The overall responsibility for monitoring and evaluation in a given department should be assigned to its chairperson or director.[4] This individual delegates to other personnel the responsibility to perform various QA activities and maintain the viability of the QA program.

The quality assurance organizational chart shown in figure 3-1 delineates the lines of responsibility in the QA Program in the Ambulatory Care Service Department of the Medical College of Georgia. Because information is shared at all levels of the organization, a clear description of all QA plan components must be written in the QA plan. Membership and responsibilities of the ambulatory care QA committee, the clinic QA committee, and the clinic QA subcommittee are shown in figure 3-2.

The QA plan should also outline the responsibilities of the individual responsible for coordination of the program. In the Medical College of Georgia's Ambulatory Care Service Department, this individual is a registered nurse with special training in quality assessment and improvement. Her responsibilities, as documented in the QA plan, include the following:

- Chairing the ambulatory care services QA committee
- Serving as a spokesperson for the ambulatory care services QA program
- Serving as a resource person for quality assurance activities
- Reviewing and recommending QA activities in ambulatory care services
- Coordinating and monitoring QA within ambulatory care services
- Analyzing the results of quality indicators to identify trends requiring further action
- Assisting staff in developing alternative plans of action based on the findings of quality assessment activities
- Communicating the results of quality assessment to the ambulatory care QA committee
- Assisting in the development of standards of care as needs are identified
- Reviewing and approving standards of care
- Maintaining centralized standards manuals
- Maintaining records of all QA committee meetings, activities, and correspondence
- Maintaining the QA plan for ambulatory care services
- Coordinating annual review of standards and QA program effectiveness
- Orienting new employees in the philosophy and techniques of quality assurance
- Recommending to appropriate persons continuing education on quality assurance
- Participating in research activities as required
- Integrating multidisciplinary studies as needed
- Consulting with persons/committees as needed or requested

Finally, the QA plan should be formally approved by the appropriate individuals and organizational groups. In the Medical College of Georgia's department this included the ambulatory care QA committee, the director of ambulatory care services, the medical staff ambulatory care committee, and the hospitalwide QA committee.

Once the philosophy and purpose of QA have been examined, the goals developed, and the scope and responsibilities identified, the organization can move on to the next step. With the QA plan as a guide, the organization is ready to implement the monitoring and evaluation process (the QA program).

☐ The Monitoring and Evaluation Process

The beginning stages of QA program implementation for each clinic included their delineation of scope of services, selection of important aspects of care, development of criteria/indicators, and establishment of thresholds for evaluation. Subsequent stages

Figure 3-1.   Ambulatory Care Service Department: Quality Assurance Organizational Chart

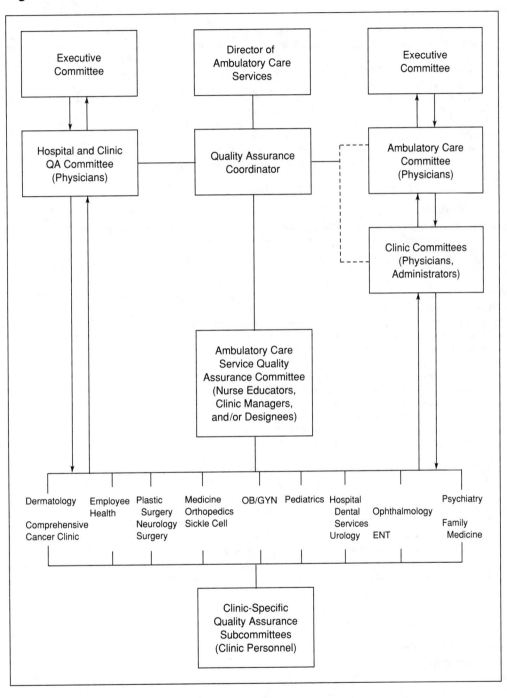

Figure 3-2. Membership and Responsibilities of QA Committees

Ambulatory Care QA Committee

Membership: Director of ambulatory care services (ex-officio), clinic managers and/or designee from each clinic QA committee, nurse educators, and the QA coordinator as chairperson

Meetings: Monthly (minimum)

Responsibilities and Duties:

1. Participate in discussion and studies on identified problems
2. Be knowledgeable about problems in practice, both nursing and multidisciplinary
3. Coordinate clinics' QA activities
4. Be knowledgeable about JCAHO requirements for QA
5. Promote QA by acting as a spokesperson
6. Participate in the development of clinical standards of care
7. Participate in the development of appropriate criteria for specific quality indicators
8. Create QA committees in each clinic for monitoring and evaluation activities
9. Assist staff in developing alternative plans of action based on quality indicator findings
10. Assist in the development of standards of care as needs are identified
11. Assist in the maintenance of standards manuals (QA, administrative, clinic)
12. Participate in research as required
13. Review the effectiveness of the QA program at least annually

Clinic QA Committee

Membership: Representatives of the clinic QA subcommittee, and the clinic manager or designee as chairperson. All staff of the clinics are eligible for membership.

Meetings: Monthly (minimum); may be incorporated in clinic staff meetings with an agenda item for quality assurance

Responsibilities and Duties:

1. Participate in discussion and studies of identified problems
2. Be knowledgeable about problems that may arise in patient care services
3. Coordinate subcommittees' QA activities
4. Be knowledgeable of JCAHO requirements for QA
5. Promote QA by acting as a spokesperson
6. Participate in the development of clinical standards of care
7. Participate in the development of appropriate criteria for specific quality indicators
8. Create QA subcommittees in specific areas for monitoring and evaluation activities
9. Review and approve each QA subcommittee's QA plan
10. Coordinate common QA monitoring and evaluation activities
11. Review and approve standards of care specific to the clinic, then forward them to the ambulatory care QA committee
12. Submit common standards of care that apply to several clinics to the ambulatory care QA committee
13. Ensure that major clinical functions are monitored, and recommend specific monitoring activities as needed
14. Review and analyze the results of clinic quality monitoring activities
15. Propose a plan of action in patient care practice based on findings of review activities
16. Serve as a communication link between QA subcommittees and the ambulatory care QA committee
17. Communicate QA activities of clinic to QA coordinator monthly
18. Disseminate findings and/or recommendations to QA subcommittees and ambulatory care QA committee as needed
19. Serve as the oversight group responsible and accountable for QA activities within a specific clinic

QA Clinic QA Subcommittee

Membership: Representatives of nursing personnel within subspecialty clinic areas (all staff are eligible for membership) with one member designated by the clinic manager to be the chairperson

Meetings: Monthly (minimum)

Responsibilities and Duties:

1. Participate in defining the scope of care for the subspecialty and identifying important aspects of care
2. Participate in the development, implementation, and evaluation of quality indicators
3. Identify major, overall indicators to be monitored that are specific to the subspecialty
4. Conduct monthly QA monitoring and evaluation activities related to patient care outcomes, practice-related problems, employee or patient complaints, and so forth
5. Assist in the maintenance of subcommittee standards of care manual and QA manual (may be incorporated in the clinic manual)
6. After each monitoring activity for a specific indicator, prepare a QA summary (by totaling criteria scores), retain a copy of the summary in the clinic QA manual, and forward a copy to the ambulatory care QA coordinator
7. Develop and implement alternative plans of care based on indicator results
8. Evaluate corrective action plans to ensure correction of identified problem areas

included data collection, evaluation and improvement (taking corrective actions and assessing the effectiveness of actions), and feedback. Each of these steps is described in the following sections.

Scope of Services

The Ambulatory Care Service Department began by identifying its scope of patient care services. This included a description of the types of patients served, the common conditions/diagnoses for these patients, the care givers involved in patient care, and the sites of care. This listing served as the foundation for all quality assessment and improvement activities.

Important Aspects of Care

Each clinic was then asked to select its important aspects of patient care. According to the Joint Commission on Accreditation of Healthcare Organizations (JCAHO), important aspects of care should focus on high-risk, high-volume, or problem-prone areas of care.[5] The Hospital Information Systems Department provided each clinic with a list of the 100 diagnoses that were highest in volume for the previous year. Clinic managers and staff selected a minimum of four diagnoses that met the criteria recommended by the JCAHO. The staff agreed on the diagnostic areas where quality monitoring activities would be focused. For example, the nursing and support staff in the plastic surgery clinic chose the following diagnostic categories on which to concentrate their quality assurance activities:

- Cleft lip/palate
- Decubitus ulcer
- Hypertrophy of breast
- Keloid scar
- Malignant neoplasm of skin

Quality Indicators

Meetings were held with support staff (RNs, LPNs, nursing assistants, and technicians) of individual clinics to select quality indicators for each important aspect of patient care. After receiving education about the monitoring and evaluation process, clinic staff were given an opportunity to define quality indicators for measuring their important aspects of care. Clinic staff who provided direct patient care, along with the quality assurance coordinator, collaborated and agreed on indicators of quality care and monitoring criteria for each aspect of care. Clinic managers were instrumental in ensuring that indicators and criteria were developed in their clinics.

Because the primary focus of ambulatory care nursing is on patient education, many of the criteria emphasized provision of appropriate instructions to patients or families. Benson and Townes (1990) have noted that a primary requirement of solid criteria is that they "must be clinically valid and affirmed through provider participation in the criteria selection process."[6] Therefore, criteria used to evaluate quality in the ambulatory care clinics were based on clinical expertise, current literature, and, in some cases, medical staff input. Examples of criteria used as quality indicators to measure the important aspect of care in gynecology patient management are shown in figure 3-3.

Thresholds for Evaluation

The next step in the establishment of a QA process in each clinic was the establishment of thresholds for evaluation. As described in chapter 2, thresholds for evaluation are

Figure 3-3. Quality Indicators in Gynecology

Important Aspect of Care:

Routine nursing care for gynecology patients

Quality Indicators:

The nursing documentation in the patient's record will include:

1. Present complaint/reason for clinic appointment
2. Patient's stated compliance with birth-control method
3. Patient's blood pressure and weight
4. Date of last pap smear and date for next follow-up examination
5. Education provided to patient by nursing staff

---

preestablished levels of performance or points in the cumulative data that will trigger intensive evaluation. This intensive evaluation helps "determine whether an actual problem or opportunity to improve care exists."[7] Thresholds prompt care givers to ask the following question: "What percentage of the time do we provide the level of care that we have agreed on?" Thresholds can also be expressed in a ratio format. According to various regulatory bodies,[8] organizations or individual departments must establish or alter their own thresholds to meet the expected quality care needs of their patients.

The thresholds established for each clinic's quality indicators were set through a group consensus process, using current literature references where available. All staff involved in the patient care process were provided an opportunity at their clinic staff meetings to define their expected level of performance for each important aspect of care. For example, the staff in the gynecology clinic set a threshold of 90 percent for compliance with each criterion used to measure the quality of patient instruction (see figure 3-3). Anything less than 90 percent compliance was felt by the group to be unacceptable.

Data Collection

After completing the preparation phase of implementation (the steps from definition of scope through setting thresholds), the next phase was data collection. Data collection involves the consideration of data sources, methods of data collection, the choice of using sampling versus 100 percent review of cases, and the development of monitoring schedules.

Because all aspects of patient care should be documented, the medical record is often the most significant data source. On the other hand, the focus of the quality indicator will help determine possible data sources. For example, patient surveys are necessary for collection of information about satisfaction.

Each clinic decided on the most appropriate timing of data collection for each indicator—retrospective or concurrent. Initially, many data collection activities occurred retrospectively, and the medical record department was required to retrieve charts for staff review. As the QA program matured, the staff shifted to more concurrent data collection (for example, observation reviews or collection of data at time of visit), which ultimately reduced personnel time for both clinic and medical record department employees. The clinic staff should be allowed to determine which method is best for them, allowing for ownership of their selection.

Initially the staff decided that rather than 100 percent review of all cases, sampling would provide sufficient information for their quality indicators. However, it was quickly discovered that sampling was not feasible for aspects of care that occurred infrequently. For example, the plastic surgery clinic's review of the nursing management of patients with keloid scars was originally scheduled for one month each quarter, with every 10th patient record being examined. The nurses quickly discovered that in order to obtain a sufficient number of cases for their quality assessment activities, they had to review every record for a 30-day period due to the low volume of patients in this category. Sampling is, however, an excellent data collection method for high-volume cases. The JCAHO recommends that at least 5 percent, or no fewer than 20 cases, be monitored for each indicator.[9] In some circumstances, using this guideline for choosing sample sizes can provide sufficient quality indicator data and minimize staff time in the data collection process.

To document their data collection activities, clinic managers and clinic nurse coordinators prepared monitoring schedules for each important aspect of care, including the names of clinic staff responsible for the task. An excerpt from one clinic's QA monitoring calendar is shown in figure 3-4.

Figure 3-4.   Excerpt of QA Monitoring Calendar of Activities for Adult Sickle-Cell Crisis

Year: _____ Data Collection Responsibilities Assigned to: _____

Important Aspect of Care	Quality Indicators	Threshold	Sample Size and Data Collection Schedule	Data Source
Nursing management of patient with sickle-cell crisis	Number of patients hydrated as soon as possible via IV fluid as ordered by physician	90%	100% review of all cases for the months of January through June	Staff notes
	Monitor vital signs (temperature, pulse, respirations, blood pressure) at least every hour and communicate to physician prior to patient's release from clinic	90%	100% review of all cases for the months of January through June	Staff notes
	Administer narcotics ASAP as ordered by physician	90%	100% review of all cases for the months of January through June	Medication administration record
	Monitor urine output during and after treatment (if patient does not void at least 300 cc within four hours after IV infusion, catheterize patient)	90%	100% review of all cases for the months of January through June	Staff notes
	Encourage oral fluids during crisis (place at bedside)	90%	100% review of all cases for the months of January through June	Staff notes
	Teach patient/family ways to prevent frequent occurrences of crisis (that is, increase fluid intake, avoid extreme heat or cold, avoid alcohol and exertion)	90%	100% review of all cases for the months of January through June	Adult sickle-cell patient education form

In the implementation phase of the QA program, all quality indicators were monitored and data collected for six months before changing schedules to quarterly or biannual monitoring. This was especially important if patient care monitoring had not been conducted previously, because each clinic needed to establish its baseline compliance rate in order to judge the quality of care being provided by its staff.

Evaluation and Improvement

The remaining steps of the monitoring and evaluation process included the evaluation of care or analysis of quality indicator data, implementation of appropriate actions, and assessment of actions. Using their preestablished thresholds for each indicator, the clinic staff evaluated the quality indicator results to assess their performance. Evaluation of care conducted by the clinic staff provides an excellent avenue for peer review. Benson and Townes strongly suggest that "peer review be actively used to highlight and validate excellence in care delivery as well as potential clinical problems."[10]

When thresholds were not met, the clinic manager or the clinic nurse coordinator (or both) was responsible for obtaining staff input to determine the appropriate plans of action. The results of quality assessment activities and actions taken are documented on a QA summary sheet by each clinic. This summary sheet might contain the following information:

- If the threshold was met, state (on the summary sheet): Will raise threshold to 95 percent and continue to monitor for one (1) month. If the threshold is continuously met or exceeded, will monitor quarterly or biannually.
- If the threshold was not met, state: Will continue to monitor for two (2) months. If the threshold is still not met, will reassess criteria, review literature, have an inservice training session, and so forth.

An excerpt from a sample QA summary sheet is shown in figure 3-5.

Figure 3-5. Excerpt from the Quality Assurance Summary Sheet for the Medicine Clinic

Date of Report: _____

Important Aspect of Care Being Measured	Threshold	1st Quarter	2nd Quarter	3rd Quarter	4th Quarter	Year-to-Date
All patients with a history of diabetes will be appropriately screened and receive information regarding detailed instruction for continued diabetic care during initial and/or subsequent visits.	90%	95%	82%			88.5%

Conclusion	Recommendations	Actions
The rate of compliance with diabetic patient management dropped during the 2nd quarter. The area of greatest deficiency was nurses' signatures on the metabolic clinic staff notes.	Identify the staff failing to note their signature and counsel these clinic staff to improve their performance.	Will continue monitoring diabetic patient care only in the area of signatures because compliance with other 4 criteria has been well within level of acceptable performance for 6 months. Plan to report data collection regarding signatures in 4th quarter 1991.

The plan of action documented by each clinic must always include a target date for initiation and completion of actions. When appropriate, the QA coordinator can make action recommendations to the staff. After considering recommendations, clinic managers respond in writing regarding the feasibility of implementation or development of an alternative plan of action.

The results of actions taken are also documented on the QA summary sheet. Those persons who took the corrective actions are responsible for evaluating their effectiveness (assessment of actions). This evaluation usually involves continued data collection of the specific quality indicators to document that improvements occurred after the corrective action was implemented.

Feedback

Communication, or feedback, is the last and most important step in the QA process. Clinic managers were asked to discuss and document in their staff meeting minutes any discussion of quality assurance issues. As clinics completed their monthly, quarterly, or biannual monitoring, their summary sheets were typed and sent back to the clinic managers for review with their staff. When monitoring and evaluation data are specifically used for peer review, it is important to provide feedback to individual providers as soon as possible.

The ambulatory care QA committee meets monthly to discuss monitoring and evaluation activities that occurred throughout all clinics. Recommendations and effectiveness of actions taken are also discussed at departmental QA committee meetings. Further communication includes the sharing of QA summary reports with the following persons or committees:

- Director, ambulatory care services
- Assistant hospital director
- Ambulatory care services QA committee (clinic managers and/or designee)
- Ambulatory care committee (includes the medical staff and senior administration representatives)
- Hospital and clinics QA committee (quarterly)

Communication of relevant information throughout the organization helps to integrate information and decrease duplication of efforts. Staff members who are actively involved in the QA process should be recognized for the opportunities they provide to improve patient care. As each step of the quality assurance process is developed, the staff will become ever more conscientious about providing excellent service and seeking ways to continually improve patient care.

☐ Initial Impact of the QA Program

Implementing the QA program had numerous immediate results. First it increased the staff's level of knowledge about quality assurance and its importance in ensuring high-quality patient care. Increased knowledge was gained from being involved in the monitoring and evaluation process, which led to increased familiarity with QA concepts and how those concepts applied to daily activities. This knowledge was gained from reading journals, attending seminars, and being exposed to ambulatory health standards.

Another benefit was improved record documentation. This resulted from the increased level of commitment from members of the medical staff and from the staffs' involvement in monitoring the medical records. In addition, the staff became more aware of patient care needs through the monitoring process. Improved documentation revealed an increase in patient teaching by the nursing staff and provided a way to demonstrate that excellent care was in fact being delivered. Efforts to implement a QA program in an ambulatory care setting are worthwhile when participants can see improvements in patient care—the ultimate goal.

☐ Key Factors of Successful Program Implementation

Many lessons were learned by the Ambulatory Care Services Department of the Medical College of Georgia in the development of its quality assurance program. The following are some guidelines that resulted from those lessons and experiences:

- Obtain as much knowledge as possible and share it (through journals and other publications, seminars, conferences, and so forth).
- Solicit administrative support and commitment initially.
- Make sure that everyone participates; quality of care is everyone's responsibility.
- Realize that the success of the program is a result of joint efforts.
- Point out the personal, organizational, and patient benefits of quality assurance monitoring to the staff.
- Get the staff to recognize the importance of documenting the care they provide; documentation is a vital component in monitoring and evaluating patient care services.

An ambulatory care organization can implement and maintain a patient-focused quality assurance program by obtaining participation of those who frequently interact with patients. The organization should examine the quality of its services in a timely and useful manner and provide ongoing feedback to the staff as well as other appropriate groups within the organization.

☐ Conclusion

Like many ambulatory care organizations, the Ambulatory Care Service Department at the Medical College of Georgia has only just begun its quality assessment and improvement process. Along with the "baby steps" necessary for QA program implementation comes the exciting opportunity to learn from the successes and failures of all parties involved. Although the QA program adopted at each institution will vary slightly in character and philosophy, the sharing of individual experiences can assist other ambulatory care groups in finding the right path toward quality improvement.

☐ References

1. Benson, D. S., and Townes, P. G. *Excellence in Ambulatory Care: A Practical Guide to Developing Effective Quality Assurance Programs.* San Francisco: Jossey-Bass Publishers, 1990, p. 55.

2. Pinkney, D. S. Hospitals may see profits drop if outpatient DRGs approved. *American Medical News,* July 1, 1991, p. 55.

3. Richards, E. P., and Rathbun, K. D. Roles and responsibilities in quality assurance. In: H. S. Rowland and B. L. Rowland. *Ambulatory Care Quality Assurance Manual.* Rockville, MD: Aspen Publishers, 1990.

4. Joint Commission on Accreditation of Healthcare Organizations. *Ambulatory Health Care Standards: Joint Commission Strategies for Quality Care.* Chicago: JCAHO, 1988, p. 38.

5. JCAHO, p. 39.

6. Benson and Townes, pp. 112–13.

7. JCAHO, p. 40.

8. JCAHO, p. 40.

9. Paterson, C. *Essentials of Quality Assurance.* Chicago: Joint Commission on Accreditation of Healthcare Organizations [printed material distributed for telnet program Aug. 23 and 30, 1988], 1988, p. 21.

10. Benson and Townes, p. 131.

Section Two

Quality Management Information System

Quality management in ambulatory health care services must rely on facts and data for process improvement undertakings. In many ambulatory care settings, the information necessary to support quality assessment and improvement activities may be deficient or nonexistent. Therefore, a first step in formulating a quality management strategy is to assess and enhance the quality management data base.

Chapter 4 describes the components of a useful quality measurement information system. The issues of data-base planning, computerization, and integration are covered as well as suggestions for improving existing information sources to increase their benefit to the facility's quality management process. As in other industries, ambulatory health care providers must be committed to securing the data elements needed for quality improvement purposes. The authors suggest long-range information management goals for ambulatory care providers who are committed to continuous improvement and knowledge-based management.

Chapter 4

The Quality Management Data Base

Patricia Warner and Patrice L. Spath

D emand by the major players in health care (providers, administrators, patients, third-party payers, policymakers, and the general public) for quality measurement data in ambulatory care is a relatively recent phenomenon. In a very short period of time, quality has become the benchmark for obtaining the competitive marketing edge. Indeed, selective contracting on the part of third-party payers has gone, with increasing frequency, beyond mere consideration of costs to include some evaluation of the quality of care provided. How then do ambulatory care administrators know that high-quality services are provided in their institutions? How can they effectively display their quality for third-party payers, regulatory groups, and the general public? Data are key to achieving this end.

A quality management data system in ambulatory care must provide certain basic information to the organization: whether the services provided meet the needs of patients and payers, whether the services ultimately improve the health status of the individual patient, and whether all customers of these services are satisfied with the level of quality received. In 1988, the American Medical Association (AMA) announced its definition of health care quality, strongly urging its members to look at quality as a number of important elements in addition to favorable outcomes. Including favorable outcomes as one characteristic of high-quality health care, the AMA believes high-quality care should accomplish the following:[1]

- Produce optimal improvement in the patient's physiological status, physical function, emotional and intellectual performance, and comfort at the earliest time possible consistent with the best interests of the patient
- Emphasize the promotion of health, the prevention of disease or disability, and the early detection and treatment of such conditions
- Be provided in a timely manner, without undue delay in initiation of care, inappropriate curtailment or discontinuity, or unnecessary prolongation of such care
- Seek to achieve informed cooperation and participation of the patient in the care process and in decisions concerning that process

53

- Be based on accepted principles of medical science and the proficient use of appropriate technological and professional resources
- Be provided with sensitivity to the stress and anxiety that illness can generate and with concern for the patient's overall welfare
- Make efficient use of the technology and other health system resources needed to achieve the desired treatment goal
- Be sufficiently documented in the patient's medical record to enable continuity of care and peer evaluation

Ambulatory care quality assessment activities must be designed to evaluate each of these parameters of quality. Therefore, quality management, when properly performed, should meet the following objectives:[2]

- Prompt attention to high-priority areas of clinical care
- Prompt development and use of relevant process and outcome indicators
- Stimulate analysis of the appropriateness and effectiveness of clinical care
- Serve as a basis for targeted education and other approaches to improvement
- Stimulate sorely needed improvement in clinical information systems
- Expand the cadre of individuals knowledgeable about the theory and methods of quality assessment and improvement

For an organization to achieve these objectives, data need to be collected from the following three areas: the administrative patient care process, the clinical patient care process, and patient outcomes. The primary data source for the quality management program is the ambulatory services information system. In addition to the elements contained in this facilitywide data system, the quality management program will need to capture information unique to its quality assessment needs.

This chapter describes the preliminary stages of developing a quality management data base for ambulatory care, including selection of indicators to evaluate patient care, identification of information required to evaluate the indicators, and selection of the data sources for this information. The issues of quality management's interface with the ambulatory service's central information system and the importance of a good facilitywide data base to support the quality assessment activities are emphasized. In addition, examples of the unique data elements needed by quality management that are not customarily found in the systemwide data base are presented, along with ideas of how these data can be captured and integrated into a comprehensive quality management process. Finally, ideas for reporting the information contained in the ambulatory care quality management data base are presented.

For purposes of this chapter, the following definitions may be useful: *Data* are ". . . things known or assumed; facts or figures from which conclusions can be inferred."[3] A *data base* is a collection of data into a system that allows retrieval of data in a manner that yields meaningful information. *Data base management* is the collection, assimilation, and presentation of data elements in a manner that provides useful information for determining and monitoring the quality of health care in the ambulatory care setting.

☐ Planning the Ambulatory Care Quality Management Data Base

Planning for the ambulatory quality management data base starts with selection of the quality indicators that will be used to evaluate patient care services. Once the indicators are determined, it is important to identify the kinds of information that will be necessary to support collection and reporting of these quality indicators. Table 4-1 provides

Table 4-1. Ambulatory Care Quality Indicators and the Data Elements Necessary for Reporting Results

Important Aspect of Care	Quality Indicator	Numerator	Data Source for Numerator	Denominator	Data Source for Denominator
Administrative management of the patient care process	Percentage of X-ray exams delayed due to equipment downtime	Number of delayed X rays	Manual tally by radiology technician	Total number of X rays performed	Radiology productivity report
	Number of referrals for services not provided by clinic staff	Number of referrals	Manual tally by health plan coordinator	Number of patient visits	Financial system report
	Compliance with nurse licensure and medical assistant recertification requirements	Number of nurses with valid license and CMTs with up-to-date credentials	Manual tally by personnel department	Number of nurses and CMTs on staff	Manual tally by personnel department
	Percentage of reports transcribed within 48 hours of dictation	Number of reports transcribed within 48 hours of dictation	Manual tally one week each month by QA coordinator	Total number of reports transcribed	Medical record department productivity report for one-week period
	Percentage of patients waiting more than 15 minutes to be seen by a physician	Number of patients waiting more than 15 minutes for each physician	QA coordinator review of patient sign-in log one week each quarter	Total number of patients in one week for each physician	Productivity report for each physician
	Percentage of patient records missing/ unavailable at time of patient's visit	Number of visits in which record is missing/ unavailable	Occurrence screening form completed by physician/nurse	Total number of patient visits	Productivity report for each physician
Clinical management of the patient care process	Percentage of patients with COPD who had flu shot within past 12 months or reason why not is documented	Number of COPD patients given flu shot or reason why not is documented	Disease index cross-references with CPT codes; chart review by QA coordinator for those lacking coding of flu shot	Total number of patients with COPD	Disease index
	Percentage of patients managed according to approved protocols	Number of cases meeting approved protocols	Quarterly chart review of different diagnoses by QA coordinator	Total number of cases reviewed	Quarterly chart reviewed by QA coordinator
	Percentage of patients with known malignancy who have weight and temperature documented at each clinic visit	Number of patients with weight and temperature documented at each visit	10 charts reviewed quarterly by QA coordinator	Total number of cases reviewed	QA coordinator report

(continued on next page)

Table 4-1. (Continued)

Important Aspect of Care	Quality Indicator	Numerator	Data Source for Numerator	Denominator	Data Source for Denominator
	Percentage of cases lacking follow-up of abnormal laboratory values	Number of cases lacking required follow-up	Copies of laboratory reports screened by QA coordinator one week each quarter; charts reviewed to identify follow-up for all abnormal results	Total number of abnormal laboratory reports identified during study period	QA coordinator report
	Number of patients seen for three consecutive visits in one-month period for whom same symptom code is assigned as their final diagnosis	Number of patients meeting screening criteria	Disease index (comparing diagnosis code and frequency of visits)	Not applicable	
Patient care outcomes	Percentage of patients developing adverse reaction to contrast media	Number of patients developing adverse reaction to contrast media	Incident report from radiology services	Total number of patients receiving examination with contrast media	Productivity report from radiology
	Percentage of patients developing wound infections following treatment for lacerations	Number of patients developing wound infection	Disease index (*ICD-9-CM* code for wound infection and visit for laceration within past one month)	Total number of patients treated for lacerations	Disease index (*ICD-9-CM* codes for laceration)
	Number of patients admitted to the hospital after being seen in the clinic within past 72 hours	Number of patients admitted to the hospital after being seen in the clinic within past 72 hours	Hospital history and physicals screened by medical record staff prior to filing in clinic chart	Not applicable	
	Percentage of patients diagnosed with thyroid disease who are euthyroid within 6 months of initial treatment	Number of patients who are euthyroid within 6 months of initial treatment	QA coordinator chart review of all patients with diagnosis of thyroid disease (cases obtained from disease index)	Total number of patients treated for thyroid disease during study period	Disease index
	Percentage of patients seen for injury and fracture that is missed on X ray by primary care physician	Number of patients treated for injury and fracture that is missed on initial examination	Disease index (patients with nonfracture injury who return to clinic within one week and final diagnosis on second visit is a fracture of injured area)	Total number of initial visits for fractures plus total number of fractures missed on initial visit	Disease index plus study results

examples of quality indicators used to measure administrative processes, clinical management, and patient care outcomes. The matrix includes the numerators (instances of indicator occurrence) and denominators (total population for that indicator) for each indicator reported as a percentage. The matrix is completed by adding the data source for each of the numerators and denominators. Mapping out data needs in this fashion provides the details needed to plan the quality management data base. Some of the data elements will be available in various ambulatory care information systems already in place; other data elements may require addition of new information sources. Do not complete the data source area on the matrix until the availability of information in existing data bases has been researched.

Existing Data Sources

Begin the search for quality assessment data elements in already existing information systems by identifying each of the major categories of information and patient care services for which data are already available. For example, the areas/functions for which data are collected include clinic visit, internal and external consultation, procedures, medications, ancillary service, recurring visit, referrals, home care, continuing care, telephone management of patient care, durable medical equipment, medical/surgical supplies, education, clinical research, managed care—second opinions, and managed care—operational flow issues.[4] Figure 4-1 depicts the relationship between the information systems housing data and the ambulatory care quality management data base. As shown in this figure, for many hospital-based ambulatory care departments there are multiple existing resources that can be used to provide data to the ambulatory care quality management program. These data range from the traditional infectious disease monitors, to billing/coding data, to ancillary usage data. Other data can be found in the risk management data base. Patient satisfaction surveys offer an important perspective of the quality of care provided, and ongoing patient satisfaction surveys that can be trended over time are a key source of quality monitoring data.

The number of data sources will depend on the complexity and size of a given ambulatory care setting. Ambulatory care providers who do not have access to the extensive information capabilities of a facility like the University of Michigan Hospitals are still likely to find a portion of the data they need in their internal information systems. Determine unique departmental internal information system capabilities prior to establishing new data sources to avoid duplicate gathering of data already available in other information systems of the facility.

After identifying the data elements obtainable from existing information systems, the next step is to evaluate their functionality. In each ambulatory care setting and organization, the specific information contained in its various data bases will vary. However, in order to be useful for quality management purposes, the data in these systems should exhibit the following general characteristics: they should be computerized, accessible, have common definitions/data dictionaries, have integrity and flexibility, and be user friendly.

Computerization

A large proportion of data in ambulatory care settings is maintained manually. With increased patient activity, closer scrutiny of quality by third-party payers, emerging prospective reimbursement, and a focus on value, the sheer volume of data related to ambulatory care can be overwhelming. A computerized system is more efficient than a manual one, less prone to error, and allows for greater access to all data elements necessary for the quality management process. Thus, it would not be too far afield to suggest that data management in ambulatory care *requires* computerization. Ideally, core data elements are maintained in the facility's central information system and

Figure 4-1. Information Systems That Support the Ambulatory Care Quality Management Data Base

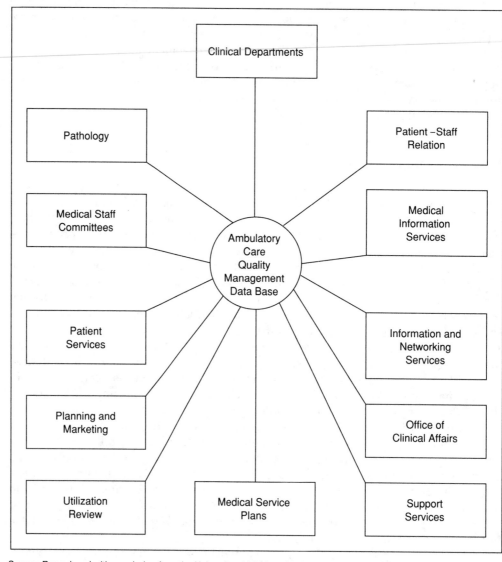

Source: Reproduced with permission from the University of Michigan Medical Center, Ann Arbor.

can be transferred to a quality management data base for further manipulation and reporting.

Accessibility

To support the quality management requirements of providers and administrators, ambulatory care data need to be accessible. Whether manually or on computer, most organizations collect and store many more individual data elements than could ever be needed for quality assessment and improvement purposes. Much of the data stored may not be relevant, and all too frequently the meaningful elements are not accessible once they are stored. Quality management professionals should define the data elements needed for measurement and reporting purposes and then evaluate the ability of the facilities' central information system to supply these elements. Programming changes may be required to enable quality managers to access the needed data.

Data/Definition Consistency

Too frequently, computer systems are established for certain areas or services that may or may not use common definitions. For example, is the term *visit* defined the same across all services? Definition of terms and data dictionaries are necessary if data are to become useful information for quality management purposes. Data definitions must be precise and convey a distinct image of the information; otherwise there may be variation in individual interpretation of the data element.[5] Explicit and objective data definitions approved by all users of the information are needed for all data storage systems. Quality management staff should be included in developing these data definitions if they expect to use the information for quality assessment purposes. If they are not directly involved in defining the data elements in the facilities' data base, they should at a minimum have access to the information system data dictionary in order to prevent misinterpretation of data elements. For example, if *primary care physician* is included as a data element in the information system, the quality management department must know whether the physician's code in this data field refers to the patient's assigned primary care physician or the one who treated the patient for a particular visit but who may not be the patient's assigned physician. Without an appreciation of the data definitions, quality assessment reports will most likely be in error.

Integrity

The integrity of the data contained in the facilities' data base must be ensured if they are to be used for quality management purposes. This requires a concerted effort to maintain quality checks for each critical data element. If the integrity of the data cannot be guaranteed, then their usefulness in quality assessment activities is questionable.

Quality control must be incorporated into the facilities' data base via edit checks in the system. A good software program filters out errors. Most errors are detectable and can be dealt with without bringing the system down and tying up operations. As a minimum, the following input error checks should be built into the facilities' information systems:

- No alphabetic characters in numeric fields
- Dates within bounds (for example, a discharge date later than the current date should not be allowed)
- Quantity values within bounds (for example, a nonexistent occurrence screen number cannot be entered)
- Direct checks against known values (for example, physician codes are checked against names to ensure accuracy)
- Consistency checks (for example, comparison of department designation with attending physician service designation)

When the program detects any of the above errors, the result should be an error message that is prominently displayed and explicit in what the operator should do next.

Flexibility

Given the rapidly changing health care environment with the major emphasis on cost containment and quality, the health care information system must be flexible. This means it must be able to take given data elements and collate and display them in a variety of ways. Quality assessment and trending require unique data displays, and users should be able to access, understand, and manipulate data to meet their needs. Unlike the data requirements of other departments, the information used for quality assessment and improvement activities may change from day to day. The quality management function requires that users have the flexibility to gather the data elements they need from the facilities' data base in whatever format is required for assessment and reporting purposes.

User Friendliness

The central information system should be user friendly. This means that quality management staff should be able to obtain, with minimal effort, the reports needed for quality monitoring activities. The best information systems have report-writer capabilities that enable the quality management staff to produce both standard and special reports and print them or transfer them to a diskette for downloading purposes. In the absence of a report writer, programming support may be a costly but necessary ongoing service.

Data Elements Unique to Quality Management

After researching the data elements already available in the facilitywide information system, quality managers may find that additional data are necessary to build a comprehensive quality assessment structure. Return to the original list of required data elements (see table 4-1) to identify the data that cannot be found or are not in a usable format in the facilitywide information system. The development of new information sources may be required to capture the data elements that are unique to the quality assessment function. For example, many ambulatory care quality assessment activities require identification of events that occur during a patient's visit. Usually, much of this information must be gathered manually through a chart review process.

One way of obtaining the data is to incorporate the collection process into the daily routine of patient care. The form shown in figure 4-2 is used in a clinic setting and is attached to the outside of each patient's record prior to the patient's arrival. The physicians or other health care providers who see the patient are asked to mark off any of the events listed on the form that they notice during their involvement with the patient. The form is forwarded to the quality assurance coordinator, who uses the information to calculate occurrence rates and identify cases requiring more in-depth peer review. Technicians in ancillary departments can also perform data collection duties. For example, when X-ray examinations are repeated, the radiology technician can use a notification form, such as the one shown in figure 4-3, to document the occurrence and reason(s) for the repeat test. This form is given to the quality assurance coordinator for data collection and reporting purposes.

If surgical appropriateness is one of the ambulatory care quality indicators, it is necessary to capture data to report the number of procedures performed and the number that met appropriateness criteria. One way to gather this information is to incorporate the appropriateness review into the responsibilities of the assisting nurse or technician. For example, the form shown in figure 4-4 (p. 62) is used by the technician assisting the physician during endoscopy to record the presence or absence of surgical indications criteria for each procedure. This form is then forwarded to the ambulatory care quality assurance coordinator, who prepares quality indicator reports and/or selects cases for peer review.

Many different opportunities exist for the collection of quality assessment data in the ambulatory care environment. By planning ahead for the data elements that are needed, the data-gathering process becomes much easier to incorporate into the daily activities of the clinic. And in most instances, concurrent collection of data during the patient care process is much less costly (in terms of staff time) than retrospective chart review.

☐ Presentation of Data

As an institution moves from the traditional case-by-case review to proactive quality assessment, the ability to track and monitor quality indicators becomes essential. The

Figure 4-2. Concurrent Occurrence Screen Data Collection Form for Outpatient Clinics

---

(Attach this form to the front of the chart prior to placing record in chart holder outside of the patient's examination room)

Physician/Nurse: Mark all events that apply to this case. After completion, route form to QA coordinator for further investigation and quality assessment data collection.

Client name: _____ Date of visit: _____

_____ Client record missing/unavailable at the time of scheduled appointment
_____ Injury to clients, visitors, or staff
_____ Venipuncture complications (hemolyzed specimens, hematoma, infection, and so on)
_____ Mislabeled/misplaced specimens
_____ Misplaced/misfiled/misidentified laboratory or radiographic findings
_____ Failure to verify laboratory results that fall outside established quality control limits
_____ Radiologic study performed on pregnant woman
_____ Medication ordered by physician not administered/dispensed
_____ Client encounter (visit or telephone) not documented in record
_____ Adverse reactions to contrast media (by type)
_____ Clients over age 50 without hemoccults performed for more than 12 months
_____ Pap smear and breast examination not documented at least annually
_____ Lack of temperature and weight documentation for every clinic visit for clients with known malignancy
_____ Lack of weight and blood pressure documentation for every clinic visit for clients with known renal failure
_____ Clients receiving more than one medication refill for psychotropic medication without physician assessment
_____ Clients who develop allergic reaction to immunization/allergy injection or drug therapy
_____ Unplanned return to clinic within 72 hours due to failure to improve

---

Figure 4-3. Repeat X-Ray Examination Notification Form

Patient name: _____ X ray ordered: _____

Date of first X ray: _____ Technician for first X ray: _____

Date of repeat X ray: _____ Technician for repeat X ray: _____

First X-ray examination not adequate due to (check all that apply):

_____ Improper patient positioning   _____ Poor exposure

_____ Inadequate patient preparation   _____ Wrong views performed

_____ Nondiagnostic quality   _____ Other: _____

Ordering physician: _____

---

reporting of quality assessment information should be concise, eliminate redundancy, and minimize paperwork. It is critical for institutions to be able to trend data and to have the capability of focusing on patterns of care or service that signal problem areas.

Table 4-2 provides a sample quality indicator report format that was set up on a computer spreadsheet program. The quality indicator data from the quality management data base are reported each quarter, and trends can be identified by reviewing the results from previous quarters and year-to-date results. Most organizations define stated goals for each indicator (thresholds). Whatever quality assessment data are reported, tracking the information to monitor actual activity and quality against institutional expectations is important; thresholds should therefore be included on the report.

61

Figure 4-4. Surgical Appropriateness Data Collection Form

Patient Name: _____ Medical Record Number: _____

Date of Procedure: _____

Procedure: Proctosigmoidoscopy

Indications Review Criteria (check all that apply):

—To evaluate chronic diarrhea
—To evaluate rectal bleeding
—To determine the activity and response to therapy of inflammatory bowel disease
—To screen asymptomatic patients at risk for colon neoplasia (that is, patients over 50 years of age, family history of colon neoplasia, and so on)
—To evaluate suspected distal colonic disease without indication for colonoscopy
—To evaluate entire colon in conjunction with barium enema X rays

—Common indications not evident

_____   _____
(Nurse)   (Date)

Upon completion, forward this form to the quality assurance coordinator

Table 4-2. Quarterly Statistical Report of Quality Indicator Data for Ambulatory Care Services

Quality Indicator	Threshold	Jan.–Mar.	Apr.–June	July–Sept.	Oct.–Dec.	Year-to-Date Average
Number of unplanned admissions to the hospital shortly after outpatient surgery	<15	12	18			15
Percentage of patients developing adverse reactions to contrast media	0%	0%	0%			0%
Number of hospital admissions following clinic visit for same condition within 3 days prior to admission	0	0	1			0.5
Percentage of visits in which patient's previous records were missing/unavailable	<5%	1.3%	1.5%			1.4%
Percentage of patients waiting more than 15 minutes to see physician	<20%	24%	20%			22%
Percentage of cases reviewed not meeting patient management protocol (different categories reviewed each quarter)	<10%	3%	0%			1.5%
Percentage of radiology examinations that required retake	<4%	2.3%	3.9%			3.1%
Percentage of patients developing wound infections following treatment for lacerations	0%	0%	0.2%			0.1%

In addition to the statistical report of quality indicator results, summary documentation should be prepared to present the results of quality indicator analysis and actions required if indicator data reveal a problem area. The University of Michigan Hospitals' ambulatory care quality assurance program has condensed its summary reporting to one form. The summary report form shown in figure 4-5 serves as the quarterly quality management report for each important aspect of care or service that is being monitored hospitalwide (including in ambulatory services). This report is used to summarize the

Figure 4-5. Summary Report of Quality Assessment Analysis and Actions

Department: _____

Division/Section/Service: _____

Infection Control Review

Type of data reviewed: _____

For what time period: _____

Number of records reviewed: _____

Number that met criteria: _____

Problem/opportunity for improvement: _____

Impact of problem: _____

Conclusion: _____

Is a trend developing? _____

Actions to Be Taken	By Whom	Target Date
_____	_____	_____
_____	_____	_____
_____	_____	_____
_____	_____	_____

Follow-up needed/improvement noted: _____

_____

_____
Department/Division QA Liaison

Date: _____

analysis of quality indicator data and report actions to be taken (if any) to the medical staff, administration, and governing board. One form is completed for each of the following major functional areas (each area may not be pertinent to each department):

- Morbidity and Mortality
- Surgical and Invasive Procedures
- Blood Usage/Transfusion
- Pharmacy and Therapeutics/Drug Usage
- Medical Record Documentation (Clinical Pertinence)
- Utilization and Appropriateness
- Infection Control
- Department/Division Indicators
- Risk Management/Claims Control/Patient Safety
- Patient Satisfaction
- Inpatient Hospital Statistics
- Ambulatory Care Statistics
- Ancillary Utilization
- Michigan Professional Review Organization Denials
- Credentialing
- Quality Assurance Activities/Issues Referred from Others

For each of the categories listed above, the quality indicator data are reviewed by the department or medical staff committee. The given service is then asked to identify any problem or opportunity for improvement, judge its impact on patient care, draw conclusions about potential improvement, and determine whether a trend is developing. The actions to be taken in response to any problem or opportunity for improvement must then be documented at the bottom of the form. Follow-up required and improvement noted are reported quarterly.

☐ Long-Range Information Management Goals

The health care environment grows increasingly complex, with tremendous public pressure to slow spiraling health care costs. Managers in the health care arena are confronted with constant demands for data and information that all too frequently are not available in a timely and readily usable format. Ideally, all the data elements needed to support the ambulatory care quality management process can be found in existing computerized data bases. Unfortunately, though, hospital-based ambulatory care settings are faced with the reality that the inpatient data needs have historically driven the facilities' information system. Thus access to meaningful data about ambulatory care is a real challenge. To understand utilization of ambulatory care services related to a given visit or encounter is virtually impossible in large, complex hospital-based ambulatory care programs whose information systems focus primarily on the inpatient admission. In freestanding centers, tracking utilization may be an easier task.

When prospective reimbursement is implemented in the ambulatory care setting, linking the visit (episode or encounter) with other associated services over time will be essential. Most organizations are therefore feeling tremendous pressure to reorient their data collection and data management systems for reimbursement reasons. This will undoubtedly have a positive impact on ambulatory care quality management programs. To understand the impact of medical care on patient outcomes requires a longitudinal analysis, including an evaluation of the continuity of care across different health care settings and frequently across multiple providers. With prospective reimbursement for ambulatory care on the horizon, one would anticipate that organizations will invest in information systems that maximize reimbursement and provide the necessary quality assessment data.

Key players in any ambulatory care organization involve the medical and nursing staffs, the medical record department, information systems, support services, administrative staff, and the ambulatory care quality assurance leadership and staff. Some organizational entity must assume responsibility for the quality management program needs—in particular their data needs. The direct care providers must lead the process with support from key departments. The prudent approach for any ambulatory care organization is to establish its data needs and then seek proposals from various software vendors. It must determine necessary or required data set definitions and establish system expectations. Then it must seek creativity from vendors, pushing for systems solutions based on integration of the multiple data systems that exist in any organization.

The bottom line is that ambulatory care information systems are sorely lacking in most facilities. Until the problems of data gathering, storage, and access are resolved, many ambulatory care quality management programs will rely heavily on manual information systems that consume an inordinate amount of staff resources and lack the sophistication necessary for comprehensive quality assessment and improvement. Until ambulatory care facilities define overall strategic goals related to their basic information system requirements, their ability to assess and improve quality will be handicapped.

☐ Conclusion

Ambulatory care information systems are sorely lacking in most ambulatory care facilities on an ongoing basis. Consequently, obtaining the relevant data needed to evaluate the quality of care on an ongoing basis is frequently difficult. A critical challenge facing ambulatory care providers and administrators is to develop data requirements for quality management in ambulatory care.

□ References

1. Caper, P. Defining quality in medical care. *Health Affairs* 7(1):49–61, Spring 1988.

2. Roberts, J. S., and Schyve, P. From QA to QI: the views and role of the Joint Commission. *The Quality Letter,* May 1990, p. 10.

3. Stein, J., ed. *The Random House Dictionary.* New York City: Random House, 1980, p. 231.

4. Matson, T. A., and McDougall, M. D., eds. *Information Systems for Ambulatory Care.* Chicago: American Hospital Publishing, May 1990, p. 81.

5. Joint Commission on Accreditation of Healthcare Organizations. *Primer on Indicator Development and Application: Measuring Quality in Health Care.* Chicago: JCAHO, 1990, p. 41.

Section Three

Medical Record Implications for Quality Review

The ambulatory care medical record must be legible, documented accurately and in a timely manner, readily accessible to health care practitioners, maintained in a fashion that permits prompt retrieval of information, and held in confidence when appropriate. The medical record is the basis for many quality assessment activities and should be the starting point for improvement efforts. This section covers the quality assurance issues related to record documentation, storage and retrieval, and confidentiality of patient information. The author emphasizes the importance of ambulatory care record systems and suggests methods by which the ambulatory care unit can assess and improve the quality of their record and record-keeping systems.

Chapter 5

The Quality of Documentation and Record Systems

Susan Dahl

The medical chart is the one permanent record of the care and treatment provided to a patient during an episode of outpatient care. A well-kept record will support the outpatient provider's claim to a high standard of patient care; a poorly kept record can make an otherwise excellent provider look bad. An organized and detailed chart allows the physician to establish a logical treatment plan based on sound reasoning and provided in the safest possible manner. The American Medical Association/Specialty Society Medical Liability Project lists the following six criteria as important components of patient office records:[1]

1. *Accuracy:* The information in the medical record should be a true representation of clinical and diagnostic findings.
2. *Objectivity:* Personal or prejudiced remarks should be kept out of the record.
3. *Legibility:* The record should be legible enough to be read by all those who need the information in order to treat the patient. Indecipherable notes in the record compromise the continuity of patient care.
4. *Timeliness:* Information should be added to the record within a reasonable time, that is, notes should reflect actual patient care and clinical findings and not the physician's memory of these events.
5. *Comprehensiveness:* All the necessary information should be found in the patient's record. The record should reflect a complete picture of the patient's episode of care.
6. *Alterations management:* Late record entries, corrections, and similar alterations to the record should be done in accordance with established clinic policy and state statutes.

Careful attention to each of the record components suggested by the American Medical Association ensures that patient records are of the highest quality. High-quality ambulatory care records contribute to improved patient care and reduce the risk of liability.

Appropriate medical record documentation is also an important defense in malpractice suits. The Doctor's Company Risk Management Department advises physicians to keep records that include a thorough and completely documented history and physical, patient's subjective complaints, objective findings, assessment, plan of treatment, and continued follow-up care.[2] Results from recent studies of why physicians are sued in cancer cases found that most physicians who were sued failed to perform basic examinations or take a family history.[3] Any evaluation of the quality of care in the outpatient environment must necessarily include a review of the adequacy and appropriateness of medical record documentation. This review begins with the establishment of a definition of the essential features of the complete and accurate medical record. All professionals in the outpatient facility should be involved in formulating this definition and should use this definition to guide their record documentation practices.

Ambulatory care is delivered in many different settings: physicians' offices, group practice clinics, community/migrant/Native American health clinics, hospital outpatient departments, freestanding ambulatory care centers, renal dialysis units, school health centers, community mental health agencies, and similar outpatient environments. Each setting must respond to varying documentation needs that result from different stimuli and regulatory requirements. In addition to federal agency documentation standards, the mandates of individual state regulations must be considered in defining record documentation guidelines.

For information about local and state regulations affecting an outpatient facility, contact the state hospital association and the state health information (medical record) association. Each of these groups should provide some help in determining how regulations affect record documentation requirements. The matrix in figure 5-1 can be used to check off which of the federal or state regulations affect an outpatient facility (add regulatory groups unique to a specific institution). Once all federal and state regulatory agencies and nongovernmental groups that have standards that apply to a specific facility have been identified, gather and compile their record documentation requirements. This list can serve as a basis for formulating a facility-specific checklist for record content requirements.

☐ Record Documentation Criteria

Many professional groups have developed record documentation guidelines for outpatient settings. Although these are not regulatory requirements, outpatient facilities should consider these recommendations in developing their own specific record content criteria. For example, the American College of Obstetricians and Gynecologists recommends the following general requirements for physicians' offices and outpatient clinics:[4]

At the initial visit, a comprehensive data base and plan of therapy should be established; these should be updated at each subsequent visit. Correspondence, operative notes, and laboratory data should be reviewed and filed chronologically in the patient's medical record. Any pertinent data regarding changes in the patient's health status or inpatient care should be recorded; this may take the form of a diagnostic summary.

The College also recommends fundamental elements for patient evaluations, which could serve as medical record content guidelines for the clinic. For example, it suggests the following basic components for the initial gynecologic evaluation:[5]

- History:
  —Purpose of the visit
  —Any present illnesses
  —Menstrual, reproductive, medical, surgical, emotional, social, family, and sexual history

Figure 5-1. Checklist for Record Content Requirements

Federal/state/local regulations affecting outpatient facility (check those that apply)	Copies of their medical record documentation requirements have been obtained		Their medical record documentation requirements have been incorporated into facility-specific requirements	
	Yes	No	Yes	No
_____ Federal Medicare regulations	_____	_____	_____	_____
_____ Federal Public Health Service regulations	_____	_____	_____	_____
_____ Federal Indian Health Service regulations	_____	_____	_____	_____
_____ Maternal & Child Health regulations	_____	_____	_____	_____
_____ Women, Infants, and Children (WIC) regulations	_____	_____	_____	_____
_____ Medicaid regulations	_____	_____	_____	_____
_____ State Health Department regulations	_____	_____	_____	_____
_____ HCFA End-Stage Renal Disease regulations	_____	_____	_____	_____
_____ State Rural and Community Health Center regulations	_____	_____	_____	_____
_____ Joint Commission on Accreditation of Healthcare Organizations standards	_____	_____	_____	_____
_____ Accreditation Association for Ambulatory Health Care standards	_____	_____	_____	_____
_____ Insurance plans in which the facility participates	_____	_____	_____	_____
_____ Other:	_____	_____	_____	_____
_____	_____	_____	_____	_____

—Medications
—Allergies
—Family planning
—Systems review
● Physical examination:
—Height, weight, nutritional status, blood pressure
—Head and neck, including thyroid gland
—Heart
—Lungs
—Breasts
—Abdomen
—Pelvis, including external and internal genitalia
—Rectum
—Extremities, including signs of abuse
—Lymph nodes

Record documentation guidelines have also been formulated and distributed by liability insurance carriers. These recommendations, designed primarily for liability control and defense in the instance of a legal action, can serve as the basis for outpatient record documentation requirements. For example, the Professional Liability Department of Farmers Insurance Group of Companies recommends the following documentation for emergency services:[6]

- Patient identifying information
- Date and time of admission and discharge
- Vital signs
- Weight of patient
- Last menstrual period
- Date of last tetanus immunization
- Allergy status
- Current medications
- Previous health history
- Results of all X-ray/laboratory tests
- All medications/parenteral fluids administered
- Patient response to medications
- Notification of proper authorities (when need to notify agencies exists)
- Mode of arrival and departure
- Notification of consulting physician and actual time of arrival
- Patient's history of present illness documented by nursing staff
- Patient history and physical completed by examining physician
- Final diagnosis/impression
- Follow-up care plan
- After-care instructions
- Disposition of patient
- Name of registered nurse caring for patient
- Patient consent
- The use of an interpreter (for non–English-speaking patients)
- Documentation of compliance with "reportable circumstances"

Another group that has been active in formulating medical record documentation guidelines are the professional review organizations (PROs) in each state. These organizations contract with the Health Care Financing Administration (HCFA) to perform Medicare patient record reviews in hospitals, ambulatory care facilities, and physicians' offices. To evaluate the quality of care provided by these institutions, minimal record documentation is necessary. The Colorado Peer Review Organization (CPRO) developed guidelines for physicians to use in charting information essential to CPRO review. These guidelines have been adopted by many state PROs and distributed to hospitals and ambulatory care facilities within their state. For the ambulatory surgery setting, the following general documentation recommendations are offered:[7]

- Preoperative Note
  1. Include with history:
     —Indications for procedure
     —Allergies
     —Significant past medical history
     —Chronic medications
     —Informed consent considerations
  2. Include in the physical:
     —Vital signs
     —General condition

—Heart and lung examinations
—Other examinations pertinent to the procedure
3. Include in the laboratory tests and X ray:
—Testing according to facility ambulatory care standards and appropriate to procedure
—All normal or abnormal results addressed
4. Include in anesthesia section:
—Anesthesia risk consideration and anesthetic planned (may be included in operative note)
5. Include indications:
—Summary statement about why it is safe and appropriate to do this procedure in an outpatient setting (may be included in dictated operative note)
- Operative Note
1. Include in the surgical report:
—Surgeon(s)
—Anesthesia administrator(s)
—Anesthetic used
—Description of indications, findings, and procedure (may include discharge notes with operative note)
- Postoperative Note
1. Include in the discharge statement:
—Any recovery period problems
—Statement of medical stability
—Person to whom patient was released, and care arrangements
—Instructions (that is, medications, follow-up visits)
—Documentation of transfer to another care setting, when appropriate

Medical record documentation requirements can also be found in current medical literature. For example, suggested medical record documentation requirements for the oral and maxillofacial surgeon's office include:[8]

- Patient data base
- Medical history
- Operative consent
- Problem and history of problem
- Radiographic and examination findings
- Diagnosis
- Pertinent medical/anesthesia history
- Review of pertinent surgical complications
- Treatment plan
- Treatment (surgical and anesthetic)
- Postoperative information, drugs prescribed, and so forth
- Postoperative evaluation

In addition to general record documentation requirements, diagnosis-specific standards may be developed. For example:[9]

- Prenatal visits, except for the initial physical examination, should include:
—Weight
—Blood pressure
—Urinalysis
—Measure of fetal development
- Charts of burn victims should document:
—Depth of burn

—Extent of burn
—Cause of burn
—Respiratory function
—Mental status
—Associated injuries
—Preexisting disease states
—Patient and family appreciation of and reaction to the burn injury and its implications

- If a patient is receiving medication for anxiety, a plan containing approximate duration of the treatment and expected outcome should be listed in the chart.
- When an antibiotic is prescribed, there should be an entry in the chart stating that the patient has no known allergy to that specific medication.
- Patients on antihypertensive medication should have lying or sitting blood pressure and standing blood pressure recorded in chart at each visit.
- Patients seen for headache should have documentation in the record to include:
—Character of pain
—Location of pain
—Duration of pain
—Associated findings
—Family history
—Allergies
—Head, ears, and fundi examination
—Blood pressure (sitting or lying and standing)

In addition to the record content, other components of the medical record system in the outpatient setting are important. A discussion of these issues follows.

□ Record-Filing System and Organization

Record documentation has a tremendous impact on the quality of patient care, but even the best records can be handicapped by inadequate record-filing systems and record disorganization. Any review of the quality of medical records in ambulatory care is incomplete without an analysis of these structural issues. If a patient's record cannot be located when needed, the quality of that patient's episode of care is affected. And, whereas a disorganized record is not in itself indicative of poor-quality care, it can give the appearance of poor quality, especially when being reviewed by agencies and attorneys. Inadequate record-storage practices and poorly organized records can lead to poor-quality care when information that is important to the patient's diagnosis or treatment cannot be found, is overlooked, or is unavailable. A chapter about quality assessment and improvement of ambulatory care records is not complete without a discussion of these important issues.

Filing Systems

Evaluating the quality of ambulatory care record systems begins with a review of the record-filing system. What is written in the record is extremely important for continuity of care and quality measurement, but if a record cannot be found when needed, quality of care can be compromised. Patients seen in the clinic without the benefit of information from their previous visits may risk having important test, medication, or diagnostic information overlooked. Filing systems must be periodically evaluated to ensure that access to information is not compromised by inefficient clinic operations. Remember also that filing systems may require updating as the clinic grows—what worked well five years ago may need enhancements today. Use the following questions to appraise the adequacy of the present filing system methods:

1. How many active records does the facility have? How many active records are anticipated in the next five years? Active records are those of patients seen at least once during the last two to five years and therefore are the records to be kept on shelves in the medical record department. An institution's specific definition of active records (whether two, three, four, or five years) will be limited by the amount of file space allocated to medical records.

2. How large (thick) are these records? Or how large will they be once the clinic is mature and has a stable clientele? Will patients be seen on an ongoing basis (primary care clinic) or on a one-episode-only basis (surgical clinic)? New (less than 5 years old) clinics or programs in the planning stage can check with other programs of similar patient mix, or perhaps a hospital outpatient department, to see whether they will estimate their record thickness or allow it to be measured. Mature programs can estimate file thickness by counting their own records, as follows: Measure out and mark one foot of file space in four to six sections of the active file. Count and record the number of records in each of these sections. Add the number of records. Add the number of feet in which records were counted and multiply that number by 12 to determine the number of inches of file space containing the records. Divide the number of records by the number of inches. The result is the average thickness (in inches) of records. Multiply the average thickness by the number of active records planned. This will give the amount of file space needed to maintain the number of records anticipated.

3. Can requested records be located within 10 minutes?

4. Are outguides used to specify the location of records removed from the main file? Are there pockets in the outguides for storing loose reports (such as lab reports) while the record is out of the main file area?

5. Is the medical record area locked when left unattended? If lockable files are used, are the files locked when the area is unattended?

6. Are record retention policies in place? Are they in conformance with state laws and precedents? Record retention is the length of time records will be maintained before being destroyed. Are steps taken to ensure complete destruction—for example, shredding or burning? *Note:* Not all clinics destroy charts.

7. Is the inactive or off-site storage area secure? Is the policy for moving records to the inactive area current?

8. If microfilm or optical disk is used for record storage, are procedures in place to ensure confidentiality of records being copied, for storage of the film/disk after processing, and for the complete destruction of the paper records?

9. Are policies and procedures for filing and retrieval of records complete and up-to-date?

10. Is there a plan for recovering or reconstructing records in the event of fire, flood, or other disaster?

11. Is there a no-smoking policy for the record area(s)?

12. Is there a policy or procedure for searching for missing records? Does it include procedures in the event a record cannot be found? Is it in compliance with state law? (For example, in California licensed facilities must report all lost records in writing to the Department of Licensing and Certification within three days of discovery of the record loss or premature destruction.)

13. Is responsibility for the records delegated? Do all staff know who is responsible?

14. Are loose reports and information filed in the patient's record within 48 hours of receipt?

The quality of records in the ambulatory care clinic can be compromised by inefficient record-filing systems. Answers to these questions can serve as a starting point for making improvements in existing record-filing practices. As changes are made, use the questions as ongoing monitors of the continued quality of the record-filing system.

Another decision to be made about record-filing systems is how the record will be maintained. A provider's ability to treat a patient appropriately, reduce risk, and defend malpractice cases is linked to its ability to access the record and the complete information therein. One record for a patient, which contains all information from all providers within a facility, will provide a more complete picture on which to base the patient's diagnosis and to develop a care plan. If unit records are not maintained, then a system must be in place to ensure communication between the separate records; for example: shared problem lists, medication lists, and physician progress notes.

A centralized storage location is recommended. Again, having all records in one place will facilitate the recording and obtaining of complete information about the patient. It will prevent fragmentation of patient data and reduce or eliminate the possibility of missing significant information about a patient (diagnostic test results, diagnoses, medications, and so forth).

Record Organization

The efficiency of record retrieval in ambulatory clinics can be greatly affected by the manner in which records are maintained. A discussion of the quality of ambulatory care records is not complete without considering the way records are filed. One of the biggest decisions to make about filing systems is whether to file alphabetically or numerically. For ambulatory care records, no one system is recommended; the choice is an individual one, best made after evaluating the advantages and disadvantages of each approach.

Alphabetic System

The alphabetic system requires little training on the part of file clerks, and it is easy to install and understand. No cross-referencing is needed to access a particular file. No systems need to be devised to verify that each piece of incoming correspondence, including clinical reports, has a number before it can be filed in the record.

However, there are some disadvantages to alphabetic filing. Misfiles occur frequently. It is difficult to establish a workable color-coding system in which misfiles are readily identifiable. The need for a master patient index is frequently overlooked, resulting in the inability to determine whether a particular patient record exists if the record cannot be located in the file. A system for indicating inactive patient records (for example, year labels) must be established. It is difficult to assess file space needs, because requirements in any section depend on the names of patients seeking treatment at the facility. There is frequent shifting of patient records to accommodate crowding in sections of filed records, based on the names of patients being registered. Finally, it is difficult to divide the work load evenly within files for more than one file clerk, in that there is no way to predict which sections contain the active files.

Numeric System

It is easy to teach clerks how to file numerically. The system provides an additional level of confidentiality for patient records because an individual must first find the record number to access a particular patient record. It is easy to determine whether a record exists because a master patient index (an alphabetic listing of all patients seen in the clinic) must be maintained. Active patient records are generally located together at the end of the files (the higher numbers).

However, a master patient index must be maintained in order to locate a patient record. A system for indicating inactive patient records (for example, year labels) must be maintained. The system requires shifting of all patient records on shelves or in cabinets after purging; inactive records will be located at the front of the file (the lower numbers). It is difficult to assign responsibility for files to more than one clerk because most activity will be in one section of files (the highest numbers). Finally, it is difficult to establish a workable color-coding system to identify misfiles easily.

Terminal-Digit System

Terminal-digit filing is a numeric system. Usually, a six-digit number is used and divided with hyphens into three parts, with each part containing two digits. The primary digits are the last two digits on the right; the secondary digits are the middle two; and the tertiary digits are the first two. An example of this breakdown is shown below:

32 - 72 - 01
Tertiary Secondary Primary

In terminal-digit filing, there are 100 primary sections, ranging from 00 to 99. When filing, a clerk considers the primary digits first, taking the record to the corresponding primary section. Within each primary section, groups of records are filed according to the secondary digits. After locating the secondary-digit section, the clerk files in numerical order by the tertiary digits. The following sequence of numbers shows how terminal-digit files would look once in place in the file area:

32-52-02
33-52-02
34-52-02
35-52-02
36-52-02

The advantages of terminal-digit filing are numerous. Records are spread evenly throughout the file. It is easy to assign responsibility for sections of files and to ensure even distribution of work load between clerks. The system provides additional confidentiality for records because individuals must find the chart number for the patient file and be familiar with the terminal-digit file system in order to access the patient record. It is easy to develop a workable color-coding system that identifies misfiled records. There are fewer misfiles than in either the alphabetic or the numeric system. Clerks can retrieve and refile records faster than with either of the other systems once the chart number has been identified from the master patient index. Responsibility for errors and misfiles can be assigned to a specific clerk.

The disadvantages to this system are the following: A master patient index must be maintained in order to locate a patient record. A system for indicating inactive patient records must be maintained. Additional training of file clerks is required because of the complex nature of this numeric filing approach.

For more information about specific record-filing and numbering methods for outpatient records, contact the American Health Information Management Association (formerly the American Medical Record Association), 919 N. Michigan Avenue, Suite 1400, Chicago, IL 60611.

Chart Organization

Organization of the patient record poses one of the greatest potential risks to the physician, the facility, and the quality of patient care because a disorganized chart may result in information being overlooked. For example, information may be filed in reverse chronological order (the most recent on top) without being organized into logical sections; or progress notes, diagnostic test reports, consultant records, hospital records, and so forth, may be intermixed. Although this lack of organization might work for patients seen only once, it would not work for patients seen on an ongoing basis. For the latter, it would be difficult, if not impossible, to determine trends in diagnostic test findings; to determine whether ordered reports were received; or to determine the sequence of events and to track patients from one visit to another in an expeditious fashion. This lack of organization may place the provider and facility at risk for liability in primary care settings.

Even when records are sectioned, the lack of clerical oversight and lack of forms design may compromise patient care. For example, in one clinic facility, the records were divided into sections: progress notes, laboratory results, X rays, and flow sheets. In the laboratory section, all laboratory reports regardless of size or originating facility were filed onto laboratory mount sheets in shingle fashion. Laboratory forms came in five different sizes—full sheet ($8\frac{1}{2}'' \times 11''$), half sheet ($8\frac{1}{2}'' \times 5\frac{1}{2}''$), $8\frac{1}{2}'' \times 3''$, $3'' \times 4''$, and $4'' \times 6''$. All were shingled onto the same laboratory mount sheet, with full-size sheets being folded in half or thirds before being taped to the mount sheet. There was no clerical oversight, and clerks frequently failed to add a new laboratory mount sheet when the current one became full. In one record, the clerks had mounted laboratory reports to the top of the form and continued mounting reports on the same form, over the previous reports. Laboratory reports were often pasted over one another, resulting in 20 reports on the mount sheet instead of the 7 it was designed to hold. As a result, some of the smaller forms were obscured by the larger forms.

In another outpatient clinic, the provider had ordered, and the patient received, an RPR (rapid plasma reagin) for syphilis. The report ($3'' \times 4''$) was returned with other laboratory tests and was mounted under the other tests on the laboratory mount sheet. The provider missed the positive RPR. For a year and a half and 10 subsequent patient visits, no further mention was made of the test, the positive result, or the test having not been returned.

Clinics cannot always control the size of reports from outside agencies but should take steps to file different-size reports on different mount sheets to preclude a test result being missed. In all cases, staff need to be supervised to ensure compliance with clinic policies. In the situation just cited (the obscured RPR report), not only had the clerk's activities been unsupervised, but neither the administrator nor the providers had spoken up about the laboratory mount sheets being overcrowded; nor had they recognized the possibility (and probability) of errors resulting from the sloppy record-maintenance systems they had in place.

The following questions can be used to evaluate current record-organization practices. Periodic evaluations of this component of record quality are an important part of a clinic's quality review efforts.

1. Is there a written policy addressing chart order? Does it specify who is responsible for setting up the charts? For reviewing charts for compliance with policy? Are clerks familiar with the policies and procedures?
2. Are chart dividers used to separate sections of the record, for example, laboratory or X ray?
3. Do policies specify who has responsibility for maintaining the records?
4. Do clerks review records for completion on a daily basis (check for dates, signatures, complete notes, and so forth)?
5. Do policies identify who may document in the record? Are full signatures and titles required to authenticate each entry? Is legibility of entries stressed?
6. Do policies specify how to correct an error properly? Are staff familiar with the policies?
7. Is billing information excluded from the chart?
8. Do policies state when administration/billing personnel may have access to charts?
9. Do policies and procedures address timely inclusion of information and loose report filing into the record?

10. Is there a committee or ad hoc group to (a) review chart forms for compliance with facility standards (for example, margins, placement of patient and form identification, use of color coding on forms), (b) review the need for new forms, and (c) review existing forms for consistent utilization and need for revision?
11. Does the facility's record-content policy meet federal, state, and funding agency criteria? For example, if a clinic is funded by the U.S. Public Health Service or Indian Health Service, is a problem-oriented medical record (POMR) maintained?

Filing-Area Equipment

There is one basic decision to make with regard to equipment for the filing area: Should file shelves or file cabinets be used? File shelves are the advantage in the outpatient clinic; like cabinets, they can be locked, they accommodate more records in less space, and they allow access more quickly than file cabinets. It is easier to move records between shelves than between file drawers, and it is easier to spot files that are too crowded. Whichever option is chosen, make sure the equipment is properly installed, safely placed, safe to use, and remains in good working order.

☐ Confidentiality and Release of Information

One of the most important customers of the ambulatory care clinic is the patient. An important consideration in meeting the needs of this customer is preservation of the patient's right to confidentiality. An evaluation of the quality of clinic record practices must therefore include the subject of record storage and the manner in which the clinic handles the release of private medical record information.

Record Storage

The first consideration for maintaining confidentiality of medical record information is that the records be stored in a secure place, meaning lockable file shelves, file cabinets, or a locked room. Secure does not mean a room that *can* be locked but is left unlocked and left unattended during the day. When records are left unattended, the file shelves or the room should be locked to ensure the integrity of the charts.

Information Release

Patients must be assured that their medical records are maintained in a safe manner and that private data documented in these records or discussed in the ambulatory care clinic are not shared with others who have no need for access to this information. If patients do not feel that the clinic is protecting the confidentiality of their medical information, they may withhold critical details that could affect the quality of care provided. The ambulatory care clinic must be sensitive to the patients' desires and design effective systems that prevent unauthorized dispersion of confidential information.

The quality assessment and improvement process of the ambulatory care clinic should regularly evaluate information-release practices. Two areas of emphasis for confidentiality policy formation and evaluation of current information-release practices are front desk and telephone requests.

Information from Front-Desk Personnel and Other Staff
The confidentiality policy extends to all employees of the organization, from the janitor to providers. Even the fact that the patient was seen in the clinic can, in some instances,

be considered confidential; this does not apply solely to mental health or birth-control patients. Consider the case of a community clinic patient whose husband called to see whether she had arrived for an appointment. In many clinics this information would be given out without a second thought. In this case, in a small community, the receptionist knew that the couple was in the midst of a nasty divorce/separation, and that the husband had threatened to do physical damage to the woman's possessions and to burn their house. The receptionist in this case replied that due to facility policy she was unable to divulge the information.

Each facility must establish a policy regarding the type and amount of information released by reception or front-desk personnel, with minimal information being the best choice. The decision must be made with much forethought and must be communicated and reinforced to reception and professional staff periodically. The front desk is an area where, all too often, information is inadvertently or innocuously released. The receptionist as well as staff can inadvertently release patient information while holding conversations about a patient as other patients are being called into the back office or are exiting from their appointments.

Too often, patients do not report these unauthorized releases of information. Sometimes they merely speak "with their feet." Consider the case of Mary K., who had finally found a physician she liked and had been seeing him for some time. During the winter, she fell in a skiing accident and injured her back. The company she worked for was extremely sensitive about injuries, having been the target of frequent workers' compensation claims. Had the company known of her back injury, it may have removed her from her position or otherwise taken action to limit her employment or advancement. One of her coworkers, a friend, went to the same physician. Some time after Mary K.'s accident, when she was well on her way to complete recovery, the physician's receptionist asked the coworker during a clinic visit how Mary's back was doing because Mary had not been into the clinic lately and staff wanted to make sure she was continuing to make progress. The coworker questioned Mary about her back and fortunately did not report the incident to their employer. However, despite Mary's high regard for the quality of care rendered by the physician, she "voted with her feet" and has not returned to that particular physician. She could not tolerate having her confidential information released unthinkingly and felt she had received shoddy treatment by the physician because of his staff's action. If damage to her career had resulted, she may have had a cause for action against the physician and his staff. Had it been a federally funded facility, the receptionist could have been subject to a fine for violation of the Federal Privacy Act. The privacy act allows for fines of up to $5,000 for criminal misdemeanors. Civil penalties allow for actual damages for an agency's failure, or refusal, to follow the act, and damages of no less than $1,000.

Telephone Requests

Another potential problem in maintaining confidentiality of patient information is telephone requests. Too often, staff are trusting of the individual on the telephone and take few precautions in determining who is actually on the other end of the conversation. Physicians and nurses are as guilty of this oversight as reception and medical record staff. A good policy is to release as little information as possible over the telephone. The first question to ask is, "Why is this information needed now, over the telephone? Could it be obtained at a later time, when the patient's written authorization has been received? Can the authorization be faxed?"

When evaluating medical record confidentiality and release-of-information policies and practices, the following questions can serve as a guide:

1. Does the clinic have confidentiality and release-of-information policies?

2. Do the policies include a statement of who has access to the records, both manual and computerized (provider staff, nursing staff, clinic staff, billing/administration staff, patients, students, others)?

3. Do the policies specify how the active and inactive records are stored? How the records are secured?

4. Do the policies state that records cannot be removed from the clinic except in response to valid subpoena, court order, or statute?

5. Do the policies require employees to sign confidentiality statements annually? Are staff informed of federal, state, and facility penalties for unauthorized releases?

6. Do the policies indicate who can release information? When information can be released by telephone, and by whom? The limits and procedures to use if information is to be released by telephone? Documentation requirements for all releases made via the telephone? Are reference manuals available to the individual(s) responsible for releasing information?

7. Are signed authorizations to release information required in most cases of disclosure? Do the policies and procedures address verification of signatures on authorizations to release information? Has the facility developed and communicated its policy on accepting photocopies of authorizations to release information?

8. Do the policies address how to respond to incomplete authorizations? Do they address the contents and requirements of a valid authorization?

9. Do the policies and procedures address conformance to legal and procedural frames within which authorizations must be processed? (For example, the California Patient Access Law lays down very specific time frames within which a patient's requests for his or her own record have to be met. Check with the state health information [medical record] association or hospital association to determine whether similar provisions apply in a specific state.) Keep reference manuals available and current to ensure that applicable requirements have been met.

10. Do the policies address any additional confidentiality provisions that may apply to specific portions of records—for example, HIV test results, mental health records, substance abuse treatment records? Are there additional measures to safeguard the confidentiality of this more sensitive and protected information? Are professional staff provided educational sessions to inform and update them about these special provisions?

11. Do the policies address what constitutes a valid subpoena? How to handle subpoenas? Who handles subpoenas?

12. Do the policies address what to do about, and to whom to report, lost records, including any mandatory reporting to the state?

☐ Conclusion

Medical record content and policies/procedures related to filing, retrieval, and confidentiality have a significant impact on the quality of care provided in the ambulatory care environment. For this reason, any quality management process in the outpatient clinic must necessarily start with a comprehensive evaluation of the record, both for content and for associated information management procedures.

The medical record is the foundation source document for most quality measurement efforts and for that reason should contain a complete picture of the care provided to the patient. Not only can patient care quality be compromised by a poorly documented record, but the practitioner's ability to prove that suitable patient care has been provided can be jeopardized. The ambulatory care clinic's record-filing systems can affect the quality of patient care if records are unavailable when patients arrive at the clinic for follow-up care. Establishing and adhering to appropriate confidentiality policies can enhance patient satisfaction as well as minimize liability risk. Without a significant effort directed at assessing and improving the quality of medical record documentation and administrative processes, the ambulatory clinic's overall quality management program is unlikely to succeed.

☐ References

1. American Medical Association/Specialty Society Medical Liability Project. *Risk Management Principles and Commentaries for the Medical Office.* Chicago: AMA/SSMLP, 1990, pp. 3–4.

2. Risk Management Committee. *The Risk Management Guideline.* Santa Monica, CA: The Doctor's Company, Oct. 15, 1986.

3. McGinn, P. R. More talk may mean fewer lawsuits, study suggests. *American Medical News,* June 3, 1991, p. 24.

4. Committee on Professional Standards. *Standards for Obstetric-Gynecologic Services.* 7th ed. Washington, DC: American College of Obstetricians and Gynecologists, 1989, p. 69.

5. Committee on Professional Standards, p. 58.

6. Professional Liability Department. *Keeping the Record Straight: Guidelines for Charting.* Los Angeles: Farmers Insurance Group of Companies, 1989, pp. 13–17.

7. Kelly, J. T., ed. Colorado group develops aid for documentation. *Quality Assurance Review* 2(5):2–3, June 1990.

8. Kelner, B. I. Office quality assurance and utilization review for the beginning oral and maxillofacial surgeon. *Quality Assurance and Utilization Review* 4(1):16, Feb. 1989.

9. Spath, P. *Comprehensive Quality Assurance: Ambulatory Care Services.* Portland, OR: Brown-Spath and Associates, 1987, pp. 17, 23–25.

Section Four

Clinical Performance

Physicians, nurses, therapists, and many other clinical specialists provide a myriad of patient care services in the ambulatory care environment. The quality management program is challenged to evaluate the quality of these services through a variety of methods and motivators. In chapter 6, the author describes the methods used to establish patient care standards for clinicians in a hospital-based ambulatory care area. These standards pave the way for assessing clinical performance. Methods for evaluating clinical performance in the physician's office are presented in chapter 7. A comprehensive clinical review program for a hospital-based ambulatory care division is described in chapter 8.

Common to each of these programs is the need to involve more than physicians in the clinical performance evaluation process. Ambulatory care providers are a clinical team, and especially in the outpatient environment, the quality of team achievements cannot be accomplished by looking at only one member of that team.

Chapter 6

Standards of Practice in Ambulatory Care

Beverley J. Moir

Measuring the quality of clinical performance in ambulatory care services requires that the facility adopt a definition of quality. This definition can be derived from the recommended standards of practice found in medical professional literature, or the facility itself may choose to set its own quality standard. The benefit of internally designed standards is that those professionals whose performance will be measured against the quality standards have been involved in their formation. Although development of internal standards takes time, staff acceptance is much higher than if the facility merely extrapolated quality standards defined by others.

Within a two-year period between late 1988 and late 1990, a multidisciplinary task force collaborated to develop standards for the provision of ambulatory care services for the patients and families attending clinics at The Hospital for Sick Children (HSC) in Toronto, Canada. Task force members were drawn from physician, nursing, and clerical staff groups involved in ambulatory care clinics, as well as managers and staff representatives of ancillary support groups, such as admitting, registration, diagnostic imaging, and health records. The standards were developed for use by all of the service and care providers working in the clinics. They focused not only on the clinical aspects of the care process but also on the entire service cycle starting with initial access to care and concluding with discharge.

At the time the task force was organized, there existed within the hospital a widespread perception that the ambulatory care services department had major problems relating to customer dissatisfaction, provider and staff job frustration, and poor morale. Many complaints emanated from the clinics, particularly from patients and families, but also from physicians. In the year preceding the formation of the task force, a new senior management team had been installed in the hospital to deal with a hospitalwide financial deficit and with concerns of patient care quality. Attention was focused throughout the organization on developing patient care standards and associated critical indicators for measuring standards compliance. It was in this climate that the ambulatory services patient care standards task force was formed. This chapter describes the approach used for standards development and the process used to develop the methodology for standards measurement.

☐ Approach Used for Standards Development

The ambulatory care setting is a diverse environment, with high levels of physician, patient, and clinic variability. Ambulatory care services are provided in many different locations throughout The Hospital for Sick Children, adding further complexity to the system. Furthermore, clinics and supporting ancillary services are administered by multiple departments in the hospital. It was for these reasons that two philosophies for approaching the task of developing standards for ambulatory care services were enunciated at the outset of the project. First, there was a conscious effort to engage in a multidisciplinary, collaborative, and highly participative process. This philosophy required that task force members represent all the disciplines and levels of workers involved in providing ambulatory care services, and that input be sought from a hospitalwide advisory group. Others were invited to comment on various draft versions of the standards; they included the patient representative and departments involved directly or indirectly with the provision of ambulatory care services.

Second, the complexity—the diversity and number of uncontrollable variables in the ambulatory care setting—dictated the need for a pragmatic approach. Efforts were made to keep the language of the standards as simple as possible and to focus on realistic measurable aspects of the care and the process of delivering ambulatory care services. Quality assurance department staff provided theoretical input associated with the measurement of quality and monitoring to ensure continuous improvement, but the work of the task force was to translate this theory into approaches that could be incorporated into the everyday language and operations of the ambulatory care clinic setting.

☐ The Standards

The patient care and service standards that were ultimately recommended and approved for use in HSC are shown in figure 6-1. The standards are comprehensive and cover all important aspects of the patient's visit to the hospital. The approach used translated into four categories around which the standards were formulated: (1) direct and indirect patient care activities, (2) services and activities associated with the logistics of managing a clinic visit, (3) human resources associated directly with clinic service provision, and (4) physical resources and the environment in which ambulatory care services are provided. The standards sought to track a patient clinic visit from start to finish to ensure that the visit went smoothly, was efficient from the patient's and the hospital's perspectives, and met the patient's and family's service expectations.

Closer examination of the standards shows that HSC's approach was to express maximum rather than minimal standards. In other words, each statement was formulated to show the maximal compliance required. Each standard included a time frame in which the standard should be achieved, who was responsible for achieving the specific standard, and how the standard was to be measured. Task force members dissected each standard to ensure that these variables were incorporated into the wording of each statement. For example, standard 1.1, Patient Health Record, was dissected as follows:

What: 100 percent of ambulatory care visits will be documented
Who: Any member of the health team providing care
When: In close proximity to the service provided
How: According to health records or departmental procedures

This approach was useful to the task force members because it ensured that each standard was explicit enough to be understood by users and provided assistance in the process of developing measurement methodologies.

Figure 6-1. Patient Care and Service Standards

Issued by: Ambulatory Care Services Policy and Planning Committee	**Effective** Date: _____
Category: Patient Care and Service	Reviewed: _____
	Reviewed: _____
Subject: Ambulatory Care Services Standards Reviewed: _____	

Preamble:

The ambulatory care services standards were developed for use by all service and care providers working in the clinics. They apply to patients and families who are seen in the Hospital's clinics, by either the multidisciplinary team or the support staff.

1.0 **Patient Care:**

1.1 *Patient Health Record*

a) 100% of ambulatory care visits will be documented by any member of the health team providing care, in close proximity to the service provided, according to health records or departmental procedures.

b) 100% of documentation will appear filed on the patient's health record by Health Records staff within seven (7) days of the clinic visits, in accordance with the Health Records Department's standards and procedures.

c) 100% of health information will be released to the appropriate referring/family physician(s) or agencies, in accordance with hospitalwide release-of-information policies, by the appropriate HSC affiliated physicians and/or authorized employees, at the time the request is made in accordance with HSC release policy (Form CO12).

1.2 *Health Care*

100% of patients will receive appropriate, safe health care by a designated member of the health care team at the time of assessment, in accordance with departmental and professional protocols.

1.3 *Medical or Other Professional Direction*

100% of patients will have a designated health care professional when contact is initiated; this person is responsible for their care while they are associated with the particular service or department, in accordance with department procedures.

1.4 *Patient/Family Participation*

100% of patients/families will be given the opportunity to participate as care givers from the time of first contact by the implementation of family-centered care philosophy.

1.5 *Communication and Teaching of Health Care Information*

100% of patients/families will receive health care information and education appropriate to their assessed health needs by the health care provider from the time of first contact, in accordance with departmental and professional protocols.

2.0 **Management of the Visit**

2.1 *Registration and Scheduling*

a) 100% of ambulatory care patients will be registered through a preregistration format or immediately upon arrival at HSC via an HSC registration system meeting all requirements for the efficient and accurate processing of the patients.

b) 100% of patients will be registered within 10 minutes of presentation to the registration staff.

c) 100% of patients will be given directions and information regarding their appointment prior to or at time of their arrival by various HSC personnel.

2.2 *Reception*

a) 100% of front-line staff will identify themselves and their positions verbally and/or with proper HSC identification at the time of the family's arrival in the ambulatory care area.

b) 100% of patients will be greeted in a courteous and professional manner by a member of the ambulatory care clinic staff.

c) 100% of telephone calls will be acknowledged within three rings through contact with clinic staff, answering machine, or voice mail.

(continued on next page)

Figure 6-1. (Continued)

d) Health records and X rays will be available to be picked up and/or transported by staff from the Health Records Department, the clinic, or the respective diagnostic areas for the clinic visit.

2.3 *Assessment/Waiting*

a) 100% of patients/families will be assessed by a health care professional within 30 minutes of a scheduled appointment.

b) 100% of patients/families who are waiting will be given explanations of any significant delays as this information becomes available to clinic staff.

2.4 *Follow-Up*

100% of patients/families will receive instructions in writing for necessary follow-up visits in time to make the appropriate arrangements. This may be done at the time of their discharge from the inpatient unit or when the appointment is made through their physician's office or by themselves.

3.0 **Human Resources**

3.1 *Selection and Hiring of Staff*

100% of staff will be selected based on HSC human resources policy and procedure and, where appropriate, based on their particular fit and commitment to the ambulatory care focus and the HSC environment. Selection of staff is the responsibility of the department head. Positions will be filled in a timely fashion given the needs of the department at the time and the qualifications of the applicants. An interviewing process will be utilized to determine the most suitable candidate. Selection committees are encouraged unless this is deemed unnecessary by the department head.

3.2 *Staffing Levels*

100% of ambulatory care areas will define and implement appropriate staffing levels within available resources and based on the demands and fluctuations of their work load. The management team will maintain a current, relevant human resources plan for the department. Human resources planning will be reviewed and revised annually. Human resources forecasting will include feedback from staff, physicians, and other members of the health care team.

4.0 **Physical Resources**

4.1 *Patient Care Areas*

100% of the examination/treatment/consultation rooms will meet clinical/service needs, yet present a nonthreatening environment for the patient/family. This will be accomplished through consultation with front-line staff and appropriate nonmedical professionals. Consultations will occur before construction and renovation begin, in accordance with appropriate codes and standards.

4.2 *Patient Care and Support Areas*

100% of patient care and clinic support areas will be maintained in a safe and clean manner. Exception reporting will be carried out by Environmental and Protection Services personnel and clinic staff on a daily basis, in accordance with Environmental and Protection Services standards.

4.3 *Signage*

100% of ambulatory care clinics will utilize signage that harmonizes with the approved signage system. Clinic administration will present all proposed signs to the signage committee for approval before they are requisitioned, according to the signage committee's policies and procedures.

☐ Communication of the Standards

The communication approach that was used successfully to gain approval of and commitment to the standards for ambulatory care services was to provide open and frequent information to various stakeholders about the purposes and approach of the task force. Very early on in the process, several opportunities were provided for feedback to task force members. Various versions of the standards were circulated to representative groups, and their reaction was incorporated. This participative approach paid off, because once all comments were incorporated into the final standard proposal it was a simple matter to secure approval by the staff and the members of the ambulatory care services policy and planning committee.

The next step in the process was to inform the stakeholder groups how the standards could be used to compare actual practice to the approved patient care standards.

☐ Methodology for Standards Measurement

With the approved standards in hand, the task force next developed strategies for measuring clinicwide compliance. Again, a pragmatic approach was desired so that existing quality assurance and other hospital evaluation processes could be used to measure these standards. There was a desire to streamline the monitoring activity so that it would be simple to use, would integrate into existing evaluation systems, and would take advantage of existing hospitalwide time frames for evaluation and planning activities. For each standard, task force members asked the following questions:

- What is the most reasonable and appropriate time frame for measuring the standard, that is, retrospective, concurrent, or prospective?
- What possible data sources exist in the hospital, that is, current information systems that can be tapped or new areas of data that need to be developed?
- Who are the most appropriate staff to be involved in the monitoring activities?

The task group decided that the same general approaches to measuring compliance could be used by all clinical divisions and departments involved in ambulatory care services for each of the four areas inherent in the standards. Further, these approaches could be incorporated into existing department and hospitalwide activities so that they did not add quality-monitoring burdens to already busy department managers and staff. The recommendations for monitoring and evaluation activities are summarized in figure 6-2 and discussed in more detail in the following sections.

Patient Care

For the patient care activities associated with standard 1, a number of monitoring activities were proposed. First, it was recommended that a chart audit, based on a simple checklist of required documentation, be conducted once a month for 10 months of the year. Clinic staff including the unit clerk, registered nurses, or physicians in each of the clinic areas could perform chart audits in their own or a peer clinic using the standard checklist. It was felt that by providing a generic checklist to monitor retrospective and concurrent documentation, it would be reasonable to expect most clinics to conduct monthly chart reviews.

Second, patients and their parents were to be asked directly whether they know who is their designated health care professional. This question would be added to an existing regular assessment of their satisfaction and experience with ambulatory care services. Clinic managers were to regularly conduct clinic rounds in which they interview or phone a minimum of two patients or families per week. Last, semiannual reports from the patient representative would be reviewed, as would the results of the annual hospitalwide patient questionnaire.

Management of the Visit

For standard 2, the time frame for evaluating compliance was determined to be both retrospective and concurrent. The task force recommended that the previously established approach to measuring clinic service times be continued. Specific clinics were targeted so that on a biannual basis, each clinic would be monitored to ensure that total service times and components of service times for their patients and families were

Figure 6-2. Task Force Recommendations for Monitoring Standards for Ambulatory Care Services

---

Standard 1.0—Patient Care

Time Frame: Retrospective and concurrent review

- Conduct chart audit once a month for 10 months of the year (that is, similar to Dentistry's approach).
- Develop a generic checklist for specific documentation that should be monitored and that could be used by all or most clinics. (Make provisions for the inclusion of clinic-specific analysis as desired.)
- Have clinic staff (that is, unit clerk, RN, or MD) in each of the clinic areas do clinic peer assessments using the standard checklist.
- Have a task group composed of a nurse, a unit clerk, a physician, and others as needed develop a simple checklist and chart-auditing process for use by the multidisciplinary health care team in all clinics.
- Survey patients/parents directly to see whether they know who their designated health care professional is. This should be done as part of regular assessment of their satisfaction and experience with ambulatory care services. Three mechanisms are recommended for this regular assessment:
  —Walk-around interviews or phone calls with a minimum of two patients/families per week
  —Semiannual reports from the patient representative
  —Use of the patient questionnaire currently under development

Standard 2.0—Management of the Visit

Time Frame: Retrospective and concurrent

- Continue to assess clinic service times using the established approach, with the next areas of analysis to be ENT clinics, hematology/oncology clinics, and neonatal follow-up clinics.
- Contact Jane Smith as a resource to further develop the expertise in other clinic settings and staff.
- Review registration data semiannually to monitor activity and to identify trends.

Standard 3.0—Human Resources

Time Frame: Retrospective and concurrent

- Because human resources policies and procedures are well established in the Hospital, it is not recommended that specific auditing be done. Annually, the financial planning process provides the opportunity of assessment and modification as necessary of Human Resources staffing levels and mix. In the future, a clinic patient assessment/work-load measurement system may be beneficial.

Standard 4.0—Physical Resources

Time Frame: Retrospective and concurrent

- Continue to use risk reports in critical indicator reporting (see figure 6-3).
- Conduct a biannual (odd years) environmental audit (preferably in the summer) using the previously developed approach and involving members of Health Protection Services, the fire marshal, a representative from Plant & Engineering, and clinic staff and providers.

---

appropriate. Registration data that are routinely collected by the Department of Admitting and Registration would be reviewed by the ambulatory care services management team semiannually to monitor activity and to identify trends with respect to patient visits.

Human Resources

For standard 3, the time frame for evaluation again was determined to be both retrospective and concurrent. Human resources policies and procedures are well established in the hospital, so it was not recommended that specific auditing be done. The annual financial planning process provided a natural opportunity to assess and modify human resources staffing levels and mix. It was also noted that, in the future, a clinic patient assessment and work-load measurement system would be helpful.

Physical Resources

For the physical resources standard, retrospective and concurrent measurement was recommended. Risk reports are routinely used in the hospital, and it was proposed that they be included in the monthly critical indicator reporting. Further, it was suggested that a biannual environmental audit be performed, using a previously developed approach and involving members of the Protection Services Department, the fire marshal, a representative from the Plant and Engineering Department, and clinic staff. Finally, the routine clinical indicator monitoring process already in place was suggested as an evaluation technique. The critical indicators focus on volume and quality measures and are used to flag areas where further problem identification and improvement are required. (Figure 6-3 presents the critical indicators that were recommended for evaluation purposes by the task force.)

☐ Conclusion

The development of standards of ambulatory care services for The Hospital for Sick Children was a worthwhile project that required two years to complete and covered a time during which there was management and other staff turnover. Once formulated, the standards were accepted by staff and providers involved in clinic services because of the participative approach used during their development. Monitoring mechanisms were developed that integrated with existing quality assurance and hospitalwide planning and evaluation processes. This pragmatic approach enhanced user acceptance. The realistic and cooperative techniques employed during the entire phase of the project were credited by all associates as having had a positive impact on what could have been an arduous undertaking.

Figure 6-3. Critical Quality Indicators

1.0 *Volume*

    1.1 Number of outpatients booked
    1.2 Number of patients who phoned to cancel
    1.3 Number of canceled clinics

2.0 *General*

    2.1 Number of staff physicians arriving 30 minutes or later for clinic
    2.2 Number of times staff physician leaves for more than 30 minutes
    2.3 Number of times resident/fellow arrives 30 minutes or later (if relevant)
    2.4 Number of times resident/fellow leaves for more than 30 minutes (if relevant)

3.0 *Operations*

    3.1 Number of and percentage of medical charts requiring telephone follow-up (excluding walk-in)
    3.2 Number of referral letters having turnaround time greater than 10 days (optional)
    3.3 Annual number of staff grievances
    3.4 Annual turnovers for unit clerks, RNAs, RNs
    3.5 Annual number of and percentage of performance appraisals outstanding

4.0 *Outcome*

    4.1 Number of patients who show up without a scheduled appointment
    4.2 Number of patient no-shows

5.0 *Risk*

    5.1 Number of patient/family/visitor/risk/medication reports
    5.2 Number of employee incident reports

Chapter 7

Quality Management of Clinical Performance in the Physician's Office

---

Paul M. Spilseth, M.D.

Evaluating the performance of an individual physician requires an analysis of the interaction of the physician's abilities (knowledge and skills) and the systems in which he or she provides patient care services.[1] Managing these considerations is the key to successful quality improvement in ambulatory care. This chapter looks at clinical performance from each of these two perspectives: individual performance and performance of the individual within the health care system. The chapter also offers ways in which quality monitoring and effective feedback from the results can improve physician abilities and positively influence the clinical systems in which physicians practice.

☐ Physician Performance

Like the employee performance evaluations common in business, periodic scrutiny and goal setting to define expected, or appropriate, behavior can benefit physicians. Feedback is an important component of the performance evaluation and physician motivation process. The greatest potential for enhancing physician performance lies in the combined management of motivation and ability.[2] Management of these components of physician performance is a foundation philosophy of the quality improvement process at St. Croix Valley Clinic in Stillwater, Minnesota, where quality assessment and improvement activities have increased physician participation, improved productivity, and enhanced overall physician satisfaction with the clinic environment. The quality improvement program at St. Croix Valley Clinic regularly furnishes physicians with information on their performance through ongoing quality monitoring and special quality improvement projects.

☐ The *Chlamydia* Study

The quality improvement study for *chlamydia* infections, completed in December 1990 at St. Croix Valley Clinic, is an example of a physician performance evaluation project that resulted in positive and necessary changes in physician practices. *Chlamydia* was chosen for study because of increasing public knowledge of this infection with a resultant increase in patients requesting screening tests. Clinic physicians wanted to know the incidence of *chlamydia* infections in the clinic's patient population, the demographics of patients with positive *chlamydia* tests, prevalence of testing practices by clinic physicians, and the economic impact of their testing practices.

Using current medical literature sources for the development of study criteria, physicians collected the following information from the charts of 116 patients who had tests performed during a two-month period:

- Reason the *chlamydia* test was ordered
- Name of the physician ordering the test
- Patient's sex
- Patient risk factors:
  —Patient less than 20 years old
  —Patient 20 to 30 years old
  —Patient over 30 years old
  —Patient unmarried
  —Patient married less than two years or with one partner for less than two years
  —Patient married more than two years or with one partner for more than two years

In addition, a list of all patients during the past 13 months who had positive *chlamydia* test results was collected in order to calculate the cost of testing per positive result found.

Results of the Study

The findings of the study are shown in figure 7-1. In-depth analysis of *chlamydia* tests for a two-month period revealed a very small overall positive rate (5.2 percent). In addition, the clinic's 13-month experience in the use of *chlamydia* tests showed the rate of positive tests to be only 4.79 percent. Prior to this study, clinic physicians had no appreciation of the impact of their test-ordering practices, nor did they have any longitudinal information on which to consider making changes in their now-apparent overuse of this diagnostic test. This quality evaluation study proved to be an effective way to raise physician awareness, and by discussing the results all clinic physicians were afforded the opportunity to change their practice accordingly.

Detailed results from the two-month study provided sufficient information to allow for development of clinic-specific patient management criteria. Study discussions held with clinic physicians resulted in the formulation and dissemination of the following patient care practice guidelines:

1. *Chlamydia* screening is not recommended during routine examinations.
2. *Chlamydia* tests should be obtained for patients with symptoms suggestive of *chlamydia* infection (cervical ectopy, cervical friability, cervical mucopus), along with the following history:
   —A new partner within the past two months
   —More than one partner in the past six months
   —No recent history of antibiotics used for treatment of *chlamydia*
   —Patient under 20 years of age
3. Patients who have other sexually transmitted diseases or whose sexual partner has a positive *chlamydia* test should be considered for testing.
4. Pregnant patients should be tested at first prenatal visit only if the patient is less than 20 years old, unmarried, or reports multiple sexual partners.
5. Positive *chlamydia* test results should be reported to the state health department.

Figure 7-1. *Chlamydia* **Tests: Quality Improvement Project Results**

During a 13-month period from May 1989 through June 1990, 772 *chlamydia* tests were done at the clinic (average: 59 per month). There were 37 positive tests for a rate of 4.79%. The charge for this examination was $23 plus a laboratory handling fee of $13. Patients spent $30,880 for *chlamydia* tests during this 13-month period; the cost per positive test was calculated to be $835.

In-depth Analysis of a Two-Month Period

Total number of tests reviewed during two-month period:	116
Total number of tests showing positive results:	6 (5.2%)
Average age of patients with positive tests:	19 years
Women tested:	109
Positive results:	4 (3.7%)
Average age of women with positive tests:	17 years
Men tested:	7
Positive results:	2 (28.6%)

Reasons given for ordering test:

Screening	35%
Vaginitis, cervicitis	31
Pelvic pain	28
Bleeding, discharge	7
Urethritis	5
Suspected exposure	2
Other	4

Demographics of patients who had *chlamydia* tests:

Less than 20 years of age	30%
20 to 30 years of age	48
More than 30 years of age	21
Unmarried	50
Married less than 2 years	39
Married 2 years or more	11

Demographics of patients who had *chlamydia* test for screening purposes only:

Less than 20 years of age	33%
20 to 30 years of age	52
More than 30 years of age	15
Unmarried	40
Married less than 2 years	48
Married 2 years or more	12

The quality improvement project on *chlamydia* tests provided feedback to the clinic physicians that allowed them to improve their abilities and skills and enhance their future patient care decision making.

☐ Physician Performance and the Health Care System

Historically, health care quality depended on the physician's doing proper work. The buck stopped with the physicians, who were trained to believe themselves completely responsible for their patient care practices. Today the clinic chart of a long-term patient with complicated diseases and multiple problems contains hundreds of test reports or page after page of consultants' reports. In following the pathway of care among specialists, hospitals, and outpatient facilities, it is hard not to notice the impact of a variety of technologies, professionals, health care services, and provider interactions. Quality management literature suggests that 85 percent of quality problems are traceable to faulty or fundamentally flawed work processes, procedures, environments, or systems—and not to the individuals who perform in these systems.[3] This theorem holds true for many of the clinical management questions that previously may have been designated as physician performance problems in the more traditional quality assurance environment. The following scenario shows how easy it is to "blame" the physician for an event caused by the health care system.

An Example of System Failure

An on-call physician for St. Croix Valley Clinic checked out the office beeper at 6 p.m., turned it on, and left for home. The paging equipment was new, and having used it once before and found it to be in working order, the physician had no reason to expect any problems with the system. Throughout the evening the beeper remained quiet, which was unusual for the clinic's normally busy practice. By 8 p.m. the on-call physician called the answering service to inquire as to why he had received no calls. They informed him that the hospital emergency department had been trying to reach him for almost an hour. An asthmatic child had been admitted to the hospital, and because the on-call physician could not be contacted, another physician was called in to attend to the child's medical needs. The on-call physician quickly checked the beeper and found it inoperable due to a dead battery. The system had failed.

The physician on call had the knowledge and skills to care for an asthmatic child. He was available and ready to take calls. But he did not fulfill his obligations as a physician because of the failure of a 70-cent battery. He anticipated the discussion that would transpire at the next hospital emergency services committee meeting as he tried to explain the event. And he could already imagine how he would feel the next time he saw the emergency department nurse who had been unable to get through to him on the phone. No harm came from this incident; one of the clinic partners filled in. The beeper batteries were replaced, and the physician learned how to check to ensure that the system worked properly.

This situation could easily be labeled a physician performance problem by quality reviewers who need to categorize such events. When there is a problem with medical care, however, physicians can be the victims rather than the cause of the problems. In the 1990s no one person can be held totally accountable for the patient care the health care system creates together. Quality improvement for groups of physicians must necessarily encompass an analysis of the systems in which these physicians work.

The Rapid Strep Test Study

In May 1991, St. Croix Valley Clinic completed one such systems analysis, the study of rapid strep testing, an antigen test for detecting group A streptococcus. The study project was initiated primarily to determine the appropriateness of physician ordering practices. The results revealed a large number of clinic patients receiving rapid strep tests that failed to show the presence of streptococcus. A summary of these findings is shown in figure 7-2.

Rather than blame physicians for overusing tests, the clinic employed quality improvement tools to analyze the system in which the physicians must practice. Using the cause-and-effect diagram as an investigative tool, the quality improvement committee (composed of a physician chairman, four other clinic physicians, a quality improvement coordinator, and three other nonphysicians from the clinic staff) brainstormed all the possible reasons for suboptimal evaluations of patients with sore throats and documented each of these causes in the cause-and-effect format (see figure 7-3). By recording each of these possible causes, the committee members were able to better understand what might have seemed a complex situation.

Whereas one may have guessed that evaluations of patients with sore throats was primarily under the control of the physician, the brainstorming exercise showed that

Figure 7-2.   Rapid Strep Test: Correlation of Results with Throat Culture Findings

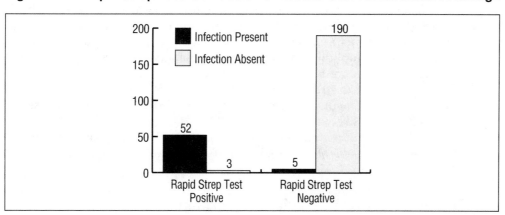

Figure 7-3.   Rapid Strep Test: Cause-and-Effect Diagram

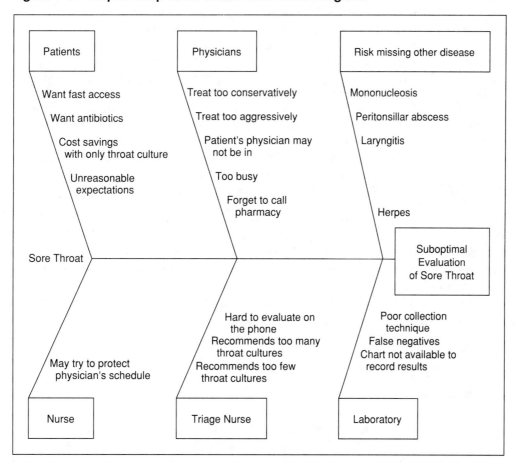

many different variables affect the management of these patients. In addition to the impact of health care professionals, the committee members discovered that the laboratory and even the patients themselves influenced optimal patient care. By completing the cause-and-effect diagram, the committee was able to focus their improvement solutions on the root causes of system failures rather than merely suspected causes.

Using the results of this quality improvement project, the following practice-related guidelines were developed and disseminated to clinic physicians:

1. The sensitivity of rapid strep tests in clinic patients was found to be 91.2 percent (52 of 57 patients with a positive rapid strep test had a positive back up throat culture). With this finding, the clinic recommended that all physicians use rapid strep tests to evaluate patients with suspected group A streptococcal throat infections; use of duplicate plated throat cultures for patients with negative rapid strep test results is not necessary.
2. If the probability of a strep infection is greater than 50 percent based on clinical findings, begin immediate treatment with appropriate antibiotics because the rapid slide test is likely to be positive.
3. If the probability of a strep infection is less than 50 percent based on clinical findings, await results of the rapid strep test prior to initiating treatment.

☐ Ways to Improve Physician Performance

Crosby outlines three steps in eliminating the waste that results from poor quality.[4] These steps have application for physician performance evaluations. First, physicians need to recognize that quality is desired and can be improved. Second, physicians must measure the current status of their processes. Third, a program is needed to correct present problems and prevent their recurrence. The effective physician performance measurement system incorporates the analysis of physicians' abilities (knowledge and skills) and the systems in which they provide patient care services. Developing a successful quality improvement process requires a commitment from all physicians in the clinic. They must overcome their fear of surveillance and "make-work" that most practitioners have come to associate with quality review activities. As the clinic's quality improvement program achieves some short-term successes, physicians quickly learn how their interests are best served by the process of review. Physicians buy in to the quality improvement process once they realize that improved clinic processes mean less frustration, less risk, and higher productivity. Physician interest is maintained by focusing on key clinic activities and patient conditions that concern them.

Physicians readily accept the tools and techniques of quality improvement because they are familiar with the scientific methods espoused by these procedures. In fact, the process of quality assessment and improvement, when described to the physician in patient-management terms, clearly shows the parallel between clinical care and quality management:[5]

Diagnostic Journey

1. Examine the process
2. Diagnose it

Remedial Journey

3. Write a prescription for what needs to be done
4. Determine a prognosis for the expected outcome
5. Treat the process
6. Monitor results

The techniques used in quality improvement can facilitate better physician performance and better clinic system controls. Many of the problem-solving ideas originated in the quality improvement attempts by private industry and can be adapted to the health care setting. Examples follow:[6]

1. *Eliminate:* Change the technology to eliminate the error-prone operation.

2. *Facilitate:* Provide the means to reduce error proneness, so feedback from the work itself conveys a message to the worker; for example, color coding for patient files.
3. *Detect:* Find the error at the earliest opportunity to minimize damage.
4. *Mitigate:* If the error has been made, minimize the damage.

☐ Conclusion

With a transition from the old methods of quality control—standards, inspection, surveillance, blame, and incentives—to the ideals of quality improvement—teamwork, scientific investigation of processes, experimentation, customer-supplier dialogue, and application of successful problem-solving strategies, physician performance improvements can be expected. There is a sense of enthusiasm and enjoyment as physicians explore and understand continuous quality improvement.

☐ References

1. Dunham, R. *Organizational Behavior: People and Processes in Management.* Homewood, IL: Richard Irwin Publishers, 1984, pp. 50–58.

2. Green, C. N. The satisfaction-performance controversy. *Business Horizons* 15(5):31–41, Oct. 1972.

3. Berry, T. *Managing Total Quality Transformation.* New York City: McGraw-Hill, 1991, p. 201.

4. Crosby, P. *Quality Is Free.* New York City: McGraw-Hill, 1979, p. 203.

5. Bader, B. CQI revisited—clinical applications. *The Quality Letter* 2(4):5, May 1990.

6. Juran, J. M. *Juran on Planning for Quality.* New York City: The Free Press, 1988, pp. 227–30.

Chapter 8

Quality Management of Clinical Performance in Hospital-Based Outpatient Departments

Emil F. Pascarelli, M.D., and Ruth Srebrenik

The evaluation of clinical performance in ambulatory care services is a process that requires a critical look at many different components of health care practice. Most health care services are provided in the ambulatory care environment. For example, Group Health Association of America reported that health maintenance organization (HMO) members make 4.7 ambulatory care visits per year, whereas fewer than 1 out of 10 members are hospitalized each year.[1] Health care analysts also find that a certain percentage of inpatient problems result from errors of commission or omission in prior ambulatory care.[2] These and other factors have created an overwhelming need for providers and payers to scrutinize more closely the clinical practices of ambulatory care.

☐ Clinical Performance Review at St. Luke's–Roosevelt Hospital Center

The review of clinical performance in the Ambulatory Care Division at St. Luke's–Roosevelt Hospital Center is comprehensive, involving physicians, nurses, and social workers who provide health care services in the following specialties: primary care medicine, medical subspecialties, general surgery and surgery subspecialties including orthopedics, ENT, obstetrics/gynecology, and comprehensive pediatric outpatient services. Review of the clinical components of ambulatory care service in these areas is accomplished through three major activities:

1. In-depth *review of events* that might signal a clinical practice problem
2. Formulation of *practice guidelines,* with subsequent evaluations to judge conformance to these guidelines
3. *Ongoing evaluation* of quality indicators to identify patterns or trends that require investigation

Each of these components of quality review is discussed in more detail in the following sections.

Review of Events

Many of the ambulatory care services have chosen sentinel event indicators of quality. As noted in chapter 2, sentinel event indicators identify a serious event that requires individual peer review for each and every occurrence.[3] Examples of sentinel event indicators that identify potential clinical care problems in ambulatory care services include:[4]

- Injury to clients, visitors, or staff.
- Hospital admission directly from the clinic.
- Hospital admission for an adverse result attributed to outpatient management.
- Venipuncture complications (hemolyzed specimens, hematoma, infection, and so forth).
- Therapy/treatment continued over a specified period of time with no progress noted.
- Episodes in which a drug that is contraindicated by information in the patient record has been dispensed.
- Physician orders for therapy/medications that exceed recommended frequency and/or dosage.
- Potassium level below normal for patients receiving antihypertensives.
- No hemoccults performed in over 12 months for patients over age 50.
- Lack of temperature and weight documentation for every clinic visit for patients with known malignancy.
- Lack of weight and blood pressure documentation for every clinic visit for patients with known renal failure.
- Lack of lithium blood levels drawn at least every three months for patients on lithium.
- No documented monthly screening for tardive dyskinesia (impairment of voluntary movements) for patients on neuroleptic drugs.
- Patients with verified hypertension (that is, blood pressure > 140/90 taken on three occasions during a two-month period) who do not receive hypertensive workup/assessment and follow-up.
- Patients receiving more than two antibiotics concomitantly.
- Patients receiving more than one refill for psychotropic medication without physician assessment.
- Missed fractures on initial X-ray review.
- Patient seen twice within one week in the clinic and admitted to the hospital within one week of last visit.
- Wound infections in lacerations treated.
- Film interpretations by the primary care physician that differ from the radiologist's interpretation.
- Patients treated for complications arising from previous treatment.
- Patients on gentamicin who do not have an audiogram.
- Unplanned return to clinic within 72 hours due to failure to improve.
- Patients started on a diuretic for newly diagnosed congestive heart failure and returned with hypokalemia. No documented diet instructions or potassium supplement.
- No follow-up on unexpected abnormal laboratory values.
- Injury of ear canal during cerumen removal.
- Bowel perforation during removal of polyp.
- Uterine perforation during IUD insertion.
- Gastrointestinal hemorrhage due to overanticoagulation or combination of nonsteroidal anti-inflammatory agents and aspirin.
- Excessive capillary bleeding or hematoma following vasectomy.

- Patient with chronic anemia seen four times within the past month for fainting spells. No workup for duodenal ulcer disease until hemoglobin is very low, and patient continues to demonstrate hypotension.
- Infection acquired from invasive procedure performed in clinic.
- Upper gastrointestinal endoscopy performed for heartburn that is responsive to antacid therapy.
- Tetanus toxoid status not documented when laceration, burn, puncture wound, or abrasion present.
- Patient with documented penicillin allergy given penicillin, synthetic penicillin, or cephalosporin.
- Swelling, pain, or coldness due to restricting cast.
- Contractures or bone/joint misalignment due to improper splinting or casting.
- Local anesthetics supplemented by unscheduled IV sedation.
- Surgery canceled because of new findings not detected by primary care physician during preoperative evaluation.
- Patient who has previously been treated in the clinic dies within 24 hours of last visit.

Outpatient departments use these sentinel event criteria as screens to identify the events that require more in-depth peer review by physicians, other members of the health care team, or both. The case review process varies from institution to institution, but generally the occurrence of an event triggers an evaluation of the quality of care provided and a determination of how further events of this type can be avoided.

The sentinel event *hospital admission for adverse result attributed to outpatient management* is an example of an indicator used by all clinics at St. Luke's–Roosevelt Hospital Center. When this event occurs, the outpatient and inpatient records are reviewed by clinicians to determine whether quality problems in outpatient care were contributory to the hospital admission. The types of questions answered during the case review process include the following:

- Do the clinic records indicate that the attending physician recognized the potential for problems that ultimately required the patient's hospitalization?
- Were appropriate outpatient tests performed and the results documented in the record?
- Was the outpatient workup timely?
- If abnormalities were discovered during the workup, did the physician document a follow-up plan?
- Was the follow-up plan appropriate to the clinical needs of the patient?
- If patient noncompliance was documented, did the physician note follow-up plans to educate the patient or change patient behavior?
- Was overall outpatient management appropriate?
- Did lack of access to health care services contribute to the patient's hospitalization?
- Did a breakdown in the continuity of care contribute to the patient's hospitalization?

When opportunities to improve patient care or services are identified during the case review process, this information is disseminated to the attending physician and appropriate clinic staff. Recurrent problem areas may prompt the development of an educational workshop for all physicians and staff or other corrective action appropriate to the problems identified.

Another indicator, used like a sentinel event but that does not meet the definition of a *serious* event, is *hospital admission of any ambulatory care patient*. Although they are not serious events because of the likelihood that hospital admissions will occur, these cases are reviewed to determine whether the diagnosis for hospital admission was consistent with the diagnosis for which the patient was seeing a clinic physician and whether the care provided in the clinic was appropriate. To answer these questions, the following criteria are used as a part of the peer review process:

- Was the patient's admitting diagnosis the same for which the patient was diagnosed in the clinic? If not, is the diagnosis something that may have been missed in the clinic?
- Does the last clinic visit reflect:
  —A comprehensive history and physical?
  —Patient vital signs within an acceptable range?
  —Appropriate medication and dosage?
  —Appropriate immunization given (for example, pneumovax)?
  —Laboratory results within an acceptable range?
  —Procedure done without complications?

Occasionally, clinics will focus their sentinel event indicator activity on specific diagnoses. For example, the pediatric clinics identified all asthma patients who were admitted to the hospital for treatment of their asthma. In reviewing the outpatient records of these patients, the pediatricians and other clinicians look for evidence of the following:

- Continuity of care
- Appropriate frequency of outpatient visits
- Appropriate prescription of medications
- Documentation that the patient's environmental factors were addressed
- Documentation of patient teaching regarding prescribed medications

The different specialties rotate their sentinel event indicators to identify cases for more in-depth clinical peer review. By periodically changing their review focus, the different specialties can ensure a broader scope of assessment.

Practice Guidelines

A second component of clinical care review in ambulatory care services involves the development of practice guidelines. The specialists define what is expected in the diagnosis or treatment of patients with particular conditions. These guidelines are distributed to all physicians and nurses involved in the care of these patients. Separate guidelines are developed for nonphysician clinical staff. After a period of time, the guidelines are used as criteria in a study of patient management. The use of practice guidelines to measure the quality of clinical management of patient problems has the added benefit of standardizing patient care as much as possible.

Practice Guidelines for Physicians and Nurses
Examples of practice guidelines that have been developed by different clinics for clinical quality monitoring are shown below. First, for the pediatric primary care division:

- Treatment of patients with otitis media:
  —Description of tympanic membranes to include appearance, presence/absence of fluid, and mobility
  —Oral antibiotic prescribed for 7–10 days
  —Hearing test performed after three or more episodes of otitis media in a six-month period

- Appropriate family counseling and follow-up when hemoglobin trait found on newborn screen:
  —Laboratory result in record
  —Documentation that provider is aware of laboratory result
  —Documentation that result was communicated to parent(s)
  —Documentation of mother's hemoglobin status
  —If mother is positive, documentation indicates partner status, or testing offered
  —Documentation of sibling status, or testing offered
  —Documentation that significance of results were discussed with parent(s)
  —Trait status listed on problem list
- Appropriate management of children with elevated blood lead values:
  —Venous samples done if micro lead ⩾ 25 micrograms per deciliter or FeP (blood lead level) ⩾ 110 micrograms per deciliter
  —Elevated FeP noted on problem list
  —Elevated FeP noted in progress note
  —Focused diet history obtained
  —General diet history obtained/available
  —Lead exposure history obtained
  —Treatment plan indicated in progress notes
  —Iron-rich diet recommended
  —Iron preparation prescribed (diet or Fe)
  —Repeat specimen within three months and within six months of initial diagnosis
  —Patient normal or significantly improved within six months of initial diagnosis

A routine gynecological "check-up" shall include documentation of the following:

- Patient age
- Gravity, parity
- Chief complaint
- Menstrual history including last menstrual period
- Contraceptive history
- Previous gynecological problems, including pap smears
- Brief general medical history including operations, past illnesses, and medications
- Allergies
- Blood pressure and weight
- Breast examination
- Abdominal examination
- Pelvic examination
- Rectal examination if patient is over 50 years of age

Return visits to the prenatal clinic shall include documentation of the following:

- Blood pressure
- Fetal heart rate
- Fetal movement
- Fundal height

Appropriate testing for sexually transmitted disease and management of abnormal results shall include documentation of the following:

- Testing for sexually transmitted diseases at indicated intervals
- Abnormal results addressed at first visit after testing
- Treatment initiated at first visit after testing
- Follow-up testing to indicate resolution

105

Appropriate management of patients with positive hepatitis B surface antigen (HBsAG) test shall include documentation of the following:

- Positive HBsAG results addressed at the first visit after the test date
- Additional appropriate tests ordered when HBsAG results are addressed
- All test results evaluated at the first visit following completion of additional tests
- Notation of impending treatment made when appropriate

RhoGAM management of patients with negative anti-D titers shall include documentation of the following:

- Results of type and Rh addressed at first visit following test date
- Significance of results discussed with patient
- If negative anti-D titer, notation of impending RhoGAM injection noted
- If negative anti-D titer, patient evaluated and treated at 28 weeks; if not, delayed for a justifiable documented reason

Management of patients susceptible to rubella infection shall include documentation of the following:

- Rubella titers below 1:8 addressed at the first visit after test date
- Significance of test results discussed with patient
- Patient given or offered vaccination during postpartum period

Practice Guidelines for Nonphysician Clinical Staff
Similar practice guidelines for patient management have been prepared by other clinical staff in the division. These guidelines define the involvement of nonphysician health care practitioners. The ambulatory care nursing staff has developed nursing-specific guidelines for areas such as:

- Obstetrics/gynecology evaluations
- Obstetrics/gynecology initiation of contraceptives
- Well-child care: health supervision
- Pediatric illness care: asthma

The public health staff has developed its own guidelines for the following topic areas:

- Breast self-examination
- Prenatal counseling
- Care of patients on anticoagulants
- Care of patients with hypertension
- Education of asthmatic patients on the use of inhalers
- Education of the prenatal patient with diabetes
- Screening/reassessment of patients in the well-child clinic

Nurse practitioners are involved in most of the physician-related evaluations involving practice guidelines. In addition, they do special studies on the following topics:

- Education of the hypertensive patient
- Involvement in patient hypertensive labs
- Cholesterol screening
- Diabetes testing
- Pediatric immunizations

- Prevention of infection in patients with sickle-cell anemia
- Health supervision for pediatric patients
- Family planning counseling

Ongoing Evaluation

Several rate-based indicators of quality provide the clinical staff with feedback on the quality of important aspects of ambulatory care. Unlike sentinel event indicators, rate-based indicators measure the incidence of an event that is expected to occur occasionally. These events are not considered to be as "serious" as sentinel events, and therefore further assessment is undertaken only when the rate at which the event occurs crosses a threshold or when data trending or pattern analysis suggests opportunities for improvement.[5]

The rate-based indicators used monthly to assess the quality of ambulatory care services include:

- *Patient access/appointment wait times:* On a monthly basis, the outpatient department supervisors review their respective appointment logs for all clinics to identify excessive wait times. The length of time (number of weeks) before the next available appointment is reported to quality assurance personnel.
- *Patient show/no-show rates:* The appointment pages for each clinic contain the necessary information for the tabulation of patient show and no-show rates.
- *Medical record documentation compliance:* This rate-based indicator monitors clerical conformance with procedures related to completion of physician orders (that is, were return appointments given and were requested diagnostic procedures scheduled?). Compliance with this indicator is noted by the presence of a (1) check-mark next to each appropriate physician order and (2) the clerk's initials. During the reporting period for each clinic, the outpatient department supervisors are responsible for reviewing a sample size of 15 medical records per month per clinic.
- *Medication profile and problem list documentation:* These indicators require the review of medical records to ascertain compliance with medication profile and problem list completeness for each patient. During the reporting period for each clinic, the outpatient department supervisors are responsible for reviewing a sample size of 15 medical records per month per clinic. The following rate-based indicator data result from this review:
  —Number of charts with a completed medication list
  —Number of charts with a partial medication list
  —Number of charts with a blank medication list
  —Number of charts lacking a medication list form
  —Number of charts with a completed problem list
  —Number of charts with a partial problem list
  —Number of charts with a blank problem list
  —Number of charts lacking a problem list form
- *Conformance with recall appointment procedures:* This indicator of quality monitors compliance with clerical processing for provider review of all medical records for those patients who failed to keep their scheduled appointments. "Appointment Not Kept" is stamped on each failed appointment sheet, and providers conduct a clinical review to determine the priority level for patient recall. During the reporting period for each clinic, the outpatient department supervisors review a sample size of 15 records of patients who missed their scheduled appointments in order to determine whether (1) the stamp was placed as required and (2) a priority level for recall was determined.

When the rate of occurrence of an event exceeds the clinic's predetermined threshold, the issue is evaluated in greater depth. For example, if the number of charts with a completed medication list dips below 80 percent in any given month, the clinic physicians and staff are required to determine the cause for this deviation. This usually requires the collection of additional information, that is, Are the deficient records all attributed to one physician or clinic staff person? Do incomplete medication lists occur more frequently in patients with a specific type of illness? By analyzing the variances that can create incomplete medication lists, the physicians and staff can determine the best corrective action for resolving this unacceptable low level of documentation quality.

□ Conclusion

In assessing the quality of care rendered by a physician or any clinical health care provider, it is critical to involve the professional personally in the review process. For example, when performing outcome-oriented assessments of practitioner performance, a properly organized study will encourage physicians to participate actively in identifying the cause of any problems noted and their effect on the patient. It is also important, where possible, to subject quality review findings to the scrutiny of peers or, in the case of a hospital-based professional, a clinical supervisor. If the study findings are discussed in an objective and nonpunitive fashion, the lessons learned will lead to desirable changes in practice patterns. It should not be forgotten that the primary purpose of professional assessments is to improve patient care. This can usually result from well-designed and properly communicated quality assurance activities.

To facilitate the overall process of ambulatory care quality assurance, it is essential to educate all clinicians, especially those in training programs, about the elements of quality assurance. Ideally, this process should begin during medical school and be reinforced throughout residency training. If the concepts of ambulatory care quality assurance can be integrated into the clinical teaching programs, then quality assurance has a better chance of becoming an integral part of the practitioner's work pattern. When this is accomplished, quality assurance will play an indispensable role in shaping the evolution and promoting the progress of quality medical care in the ambulatory care setting.

□ References

1. Group Health Association of America. *HMO Industry Profile.* Vol. 2, *Utilization Patterns.* Washington, DC: GHAA, 1988.

2. Joint Commission on Accreditation of Healthcare Organizations. *Quality Assurance in Managed Care.* Chicago: JCAHO, 1989, p. 20.

3. Joint Commission on Accreditation of Healthcare Organizations. *Primer on Indicator Development and Application.* Chicago: JCAHO, 1990, p. 11.

4. Spath, P. *Hospital Quality Indicator Workbook.* Portland: Brown-Spath and Associates, 1989, p. 37.

5. Joint Commission on Accreditation of Healthcare Organizations. *Primer on Indicator Development and Application.* Chicago: JCAHO, 1990, p. 11.

Section Five

Continuity of Health Care Services

In no other environment is continuity of care so critical as it is in ambulatory care. Continuity is essential for care of complex cases with multiple diagnoses, for well-baby care and other preventive measures, and for treatment of substance abuse, depressive disorders, chronic illness, cancer, and so forth. Timely and appropriate linkages between primary and specialty care, coordination among specialists, appropriate combinations of medications prescribed, and the coordinated use of ancillary services are indicators of care continuity. In addition, as a patient requires different levels of care, coordination of his or her health care needs with different providers must be timely as well as orderly. Ensuring continuity of care for the individual patient is a challenge for the ambulatory care quality management program. Equally challenging is the retrospective evaluation of system malfunctions that affect continuity.

In this section, the methods for assessing the quality of patient care continuity are presented from two different perspectives—a managed care setting and a hospital-based ambulatory care provider. Fundamental issues, such as what to measure, how to collect data, how to display quality assessment findings, and the goals of continuity-of-care evaluations, are discussed.

Chapter 9

Continuity of Care in a Managed Care Program

Pam Blackmore

Continuity of health care refers to the continuous flow of care in a timely and appropriate manner. It includes preventive services, linkages between primary and specialty care, coordination among specialists, appropriate combinations of prescribed medication, coordinated use of ancillary services, and timely placement at different levels of care. Good continuity of care is characterized by sustained, uninterrupted professional service(s) rendered to a single patient by one or more physicians or other providers for a single episode of illness or a series of illnesses during which the provider(s) coordinates communication and utilization of health care services.

As the volume of health care services shifts to the ambulatory care setting, health systems and health plans must have mechanisms in place to ensure that patients receive timely, continuous, and appropriate initial and follow-up health care services. Review of the quality of continuity of care is an essential component of a clinic's or health plan's quality management program. Several mechanisms are available to clinics and managed care health plans to assess continuity of care. These include patient and provider feedback, evaluation of compliance with referral management protocols and specific contractual requirements, and focused studies of encounter/paid claims data, medical record protocols, preventive care standards, and patient reminders. As one of two chapters on measuring and ensuring continuity of care, this chapter focuses on the health plan's perspective of quality management.

☐ Measuring Continuity of Care

Federally approved health maintenance organizations (HMOs) and competitive medical plans are required to have a system in place to ensure continuity of care among providers.[1] Documentation of compliance with this requirement necessitates periodic quality review of continuity issues. Several different measures or indicators of quality can be used to evaluate continuity. For example, the health plan may choose to define diagnosis- or condition-specific measures of continuity, focusing on high-volume, high-risk, or problem-prone areas of patient care. Patient and provider complaints or grievances and satisfaction surveys are another potential source of information related to continuity. The health plan's billing/encounter data can help in targeting areas for special studies related to continuity of care. The federal and state regulations governing health plans and their commitment to continuity of services may be a source of quality indicator ideas. Information collected from risk management reports and review of legal claims data may also uncover system problems. The information included in the health plan's formal quality management program may serve as a springboard for continuity-of-care measures. Ideally, all of the information related to quality of care is entered into a common data base for reporting and review of trends, some of which may illustrate continuity-of-care issues.

Suggested indicator screens that assist in measuring the quality of continuity of care include the following:

- The number of patients developing drug overdose/toxicity (that is, adverse drug reactions, untoward effects related to concomitant medication usage—for example, the use of Cimetidine and Famotidine simultaneously)
- Inadequate medical record documentation:
  —Lack of referral/consultation records: Written report should be received within seven working days after date of service, or verbal contact should be made immediately for emergency situations
  —Lack of emergency records: Written report should be received within seven working days after date of service, or verbal contact should be made immediately for emergency situations
  —Lack of ancillary services reports: Written report should be received within seven working days after date of service, or verbal contact should be made immediately for emergency situations or to report critical values
  —Lack of immunization records
  —Lack of allergy documentation
  —Lack of patient notification of treatment and testing results, or underuse of appropriate referrals/consultations
  —Lack of patient instruction on preventive care standards
- Patient noncompliance:
  —Three missed appointments per year
  —Two missed appointments in one month
- Delay in treatment or diagnosis resulting in adverse occurrence
- Lack of preventive care:
  —Prenatal visits
  —Well-baby visits
  —Periodic examinations
  —Mammography
  —Pap smears
- Out-of-area services greater than 10 percent of overall health care costs
- Patients receiving duplicate medications from different providers
- Diagnosis- or condition-specific issues:
  —Complete blood count not performed within 30 days of a diagnosis of infectious mononucleosis
  —Chest X ray not performed within two weeks of a patient's positive intermediate purified protein derivative (PPD) test
  —Fundus examination not performed annually for patients with confirmed diagnosis of diabetes; no ophthalmologist referral when retinopathy is found
  —Patients with iron deficiency anemia not given a repeat hemoglobin or hematocrit four to six weeks after hemoglobin or hematocrit value is normal
  —Anticoagulants prescribed within 45 days following episode of gastrointestinal bleeding
  —Folate level not done at least yearly for patients receiving phenytoin (Dilantin)

—Blood urea nitrogen (BUN) and/or creatinine, potassium, and uric acid not done at least yearly for hypertensive patients receiving diuretics

—Sedative-hypnotics, narcotics, or antihistamines prescribed for patients with chronic obstructive pulmonary disease

—For a child sustaining more than two injuries, accidents, and/or poisonings in one year, no record indicating an inquiry or referral concerning the possibility of child abuse

—For patients over the age of 45 with a urine test positive for protein or occult blood, no evidence of a rectal examination with stool guaiac test within 12 months

☐ Continuity-of-Care Standards

Acceptable continuity-of-care standards should include both general care and prevention.

General Care Standards

A definition of acceptable continuity of care must be specified by the health plan and included in the contracts made with individual health care providers. Clear and specific provider contract language can set the standard of care and ground rules for referral services, specifically addressing the health plan's commitment to continuity of care. Acceptable continuity of care and specific contract language can be developed for each type of health care service, ranging from laboratory to specialty services. For example, the contract for specialist providers may include the following entry: "Specialist shall provide a written record regarding all patient encounters. This shall include submission of a report or communication to the referring provider after the initial referral or as necessary/requested during follow-up care." The health plan might also consider adopting the requirement of the Accreditation Association for Ambulatory Health Care (AAAHC) standards for pathology and medical laboratory services, which states that test results be distributed within 24 hours after completion of a test and copies of the results be maintained in the laboratory.[2] These standards would be incorporated into the contracts with laboratory services. Contracts with emergency rooms and clinics might include the health plan's standard that a written report shall be submitted to the patient's primary care provider within a specified number of working days after delivering emergency services.

Following are other examples of continuity-of-care standards that might be adopted by the health plan and communicated to all plan providers:

- Referral services information must be communicated immediately by the health plan in situations requiring emergency intervention (additional testing, referral, or hospitalization).
- Teleconferences between providers used to discuss diagnostic testing results, consultation, or treatments should be followed up with a written report or annotation in the patient chart.
- All specialty and primary health care providers must maintain hospital privileges or have an agreement with a provider to accept their patients if hospitalization becomes necessary.

The continuity-of-care standards established by the health plan and written into each provider's contract serve as the plan's definition of quality for patient care continuity. These standards form the basis for later review and evaluation to ensure that the health plan and its providers continue to maintain at least this minimal acceptable level of quality.

Preventive Care Standards

Another aspect of health care continuity is preventive care. The HMO must establish preventive care standards and disseminate these requirements to all primary care providers. The HMO should adopt as their preventive care standards those guidelines already established by such groups as the American Cancer Society, the U.S. Public Health Department's Preventive Services Task Force, and the professional societies of each medical specialty. For example, the American Cancer Society and the National Cancer Institute have defined and disseminated recommendations for the frequency of cancer detection examinations (stool occult-blood test, rectal examination, sigmoidoscopy, Papanicolaou's (pap) smear, pelvic examination, breast examination, and mammography).[3-6] The U.S. Public Health Department has defined standards for well-baby and routine adult preventive care.[7]

The health plan's preventive standards should be based on those established by medical professional groups and societies. Once standards have been defined, the health plan can compare their plan members' preventive care experience with these standards. In evaluating compliance with preventive care guidelines, the health plan must consider that not all patients will obtain their preventive care through the health plan providers. For example, some patients with dual health coverage may select a provider for pap smears and mammography that is not a member of their personal health plan; other patients may use county health clinics or choose to pay for services out-of-pocket. In measuring compliance with preventive standards, these variables must be considered by the health plan and the study's data collection adjusted accordingly.

Another component of preventive care is education. Providers must spend time with the patient, giving verbal instruction on preventive care as well as written documentation to enhance the members' learning process. The HMO should require that all such instructions be documented in the medical record to enable retrospective review of compliance with preventive care education requirements.

☐ Effect of Patient Noncompliance on Continuity of Care

Patients must assume some responsibility for the success or failure of their health care. Patients who fail to follow recommended treatment plans, fail to show up for appointments, or refuse diagnostic studies and treatment will circumvent all efforts to ensure continuity of care. It is helpful for the health plan to assess their current rate of patient compliance, that is, missed appointments and lack of preventive care, and compare this information to previous years. The health plan should consider contacting members/patients with more than three missed appointments per year, or more than two missed appointments in one month. Personal contact by health plan staff may have a positive impact on the patient's future health care involvement and ensure continuity for preventive services.

Due to the time-consuming nature of such a project, it is recommended that the plan conduct a review of available data that already have been collected regarding patient noncompliance, that is, failed appointments and patient refusal to follow recommended treatment plans. In the absence of such data, it is advisable to begin the patient compliance monitoring program on a small scale, by conducting a preliminary review to determine appropriateness and effectiveness. The program can then be implemented on a wider scale.

☐ Study Methodologies

The health plan has several options for studying continuity-of-care issues. The choice of study methodologies will depend largely on the staffing levels of the health plan's quality management department and the availability of computerized information. In general, continuity of care can be measured through five different techniques: surveys, focused studies, review of complaints and grievances, case reviews, and medical record reviews.

Provider/Patient Surveys

Surveying providers and patients is a good way to assess their perception about continuity of care. These surveys should be released on a regular basis (preferably annually). Surveys should include questions that allow provider/patient feedback on appointment waiting times for primary or specialty care, and provider communication to the patient/member regarding diagnostic testing, test results, suggested treatments, preventive care suggestions, or referrals/consultations.

Cost savings can be maximized if the survey combines many different quality measures—accessibility, continuity of care, management appropriateness, clinic staff satisfaction, and overall contentment with the health plan. This method is preferred over release of multiple surveys addressing related issues. If continuity problem areas are identified through this general survey process, more detailed studies can then be initiated. In addition, provider and member telephone interviews and one-on-one personal interviews or written questionnaires can be very helpful. Surveys are also useful methods for determining whether action plans for improvement were successful in having a positive impact on continuity.

Examples of patient survey questions related to continuity of care are shown in figure 9-1. Questions for physicians and other providers are shown in figure 9-2. These surveys are intended to be part of a larger study, with the questions shown in the figures addressing only continuity issues. Demographic information including age, sex, and ambulatory care organization information should also be included on the survey, as well as space for comments and a phone number or address where respondents may contact the organization directly for comments or complaints, or to express satisfaction.

Focused Studies

Studies of a particular topic, that is, diagnosis, condition, medication, and so forth, are another mechanism for monitoring continuity of care. For example, a health plan may choose to review laboratory services to determine whether laboratory results have been communicated to the referring provider within 24 hours (or immediately for critical values). Ideally, there are contractual requirements for these performance standards, but focused studies allow the health plan to measure contract compliance or develop an acceptable threshold that is realistic and appropriate for the service. Performance standards should be based on accepted medical literature references, clinical practice standards developed by medical professional societies, or the standard of practice exhibited by current plan providers. Study topics might include time required to receive diagnostic testing results, preventive care compliance, receipt of referral/consultation notes, and patients receiving identical medications from different providers. Information to conduct a focused study may be collected from several sources—claims/encounter data, complaints and grievances, or QM case reviews.

Complaints and Grievances

Although patient complaints and grievances related to quality of care may not constitute the major driving force behind identification and improvement of continuity-of-care

Figure 9-1. Continuity-of-Care Questions for Patients

1. How many times did you see your primary care provider (the physician you selected for your routine care)?

   _____ Within the past month
   _____ Within the past 6 months
   _____ Within the past year
   _____ Longer than one year ago

2. Did your primary care provider refer you to other providers in the past year?

   Yes _____   No _____

3. If "Yes" to #2: When you were referred to a provider, did he or she have information on your case prior to your visit?

   Yes _____   No _____

4. Were you notified of your testing, treatments, or consultation results by your primary or specialty provider?

   Yes _____   No _____

5. Were your health care services ever delayed due to lack of information or a delay in testing results?

   Yes _____   No _____

   If yes, please explain:

6. Did you change your primary care provider in the past year?

   Yes _____   No _____

7. If "Yes" to #6: Did you sign a release for your medical records so they could be forwarded to your new primary care provider?

   Yes _____   No _____

8. If "Yes" to #7: Did the new primary care provider have your medical information when you visited him or her after signing the release?

   Yes _____   No _____

9. Has your primary care provider recommended any measures you should take to improve your health (check those that apply)?

Exercise instructions?	Yes _____	No _____
Dietary advice?	Yes _____	No _____
Stop-smoking instructions?	Yes _____	No _____
Alcohol intake advice?	Yes _____	No _____
Recommended testing (that is, mammogram, stool for occult blood, pap smear, EKG)?	Yes _____	No _____
Recommend treatments (that is, immunizations)	Yes _____	No _____
Other	Yes _____	No _____
(please provide details below)		

10. If "Yes" to any questions in #9: Did you follow the provider's recommendations?

    Yes _____   No _____

11. Were return visits to your primary provider or another provider recommended during your last visit to your primary provider?

    Yes _____   No _____

12. If you answered "Yes" to #11: Did you see the provider as recommended?

    Yes _____   No _____

Figure 9-2. Continuity-of-Care Questions for Providers

---

1. Were referrals available to the health plan members in a timely manner?

   Yes _____   No _____

2. Were the results of consultations, testing, or treatments communicated to you in a timely manner?

   Yes _____   No _____

3. Has patient treatment ever been delayed due to lack of information from other providers?

   Yes _____   No _____

4. Are there any contracting providers you refuse to refer your patients to because of lack of continuity of care, that is, test results received late or not at all, or the provider's failure to notify you of consultation findings?

   Yes _____   No _____

   Optional: If "yes" to #4: please list those providers you no longer use as referrals, and why:

   _____

   _____

   _____

---

issues, the absence of a mechanism to address them would surely cause the health plan members to believe the health plan was not responsive to their needs. Categorizing grievances by type of issue, that is, continuity of care, will assist in the process of evaluating that factor. Final review and tracking of quality of care grievances should be the responsibility of the quality management department staff, allowing this department an opportunity to evaluate the continuity of care and identify trends accurately. The number of complaints and grievances per total plan participants should be used to compare current year results with prior year results. Grievances related to the continuity of care should be tracked so that the information can be reported separately. This is necessary to measure the effects of those aspects of the quality-of-care program that are designed to identify and improve the continuity of care.

Case Reviews

Quality-of-care and risk-management case reviews will also provide information on continuity, particularly if this information is categorized in such a way as to identify continuity-of-care problems as separate issues. Conversely, information obtained through other quality measures may help in the selection of cases for review. For example, when studying providers' compliance with the specialty referral requirements of the HMO, health plan staff might identify providers who unknowingly fail to contact patients with the results of laboratory examinations. Continuity-of-care issues may also be identified by other health plan departments. For example, provider services personnel might receive complaints from physician office staff that patients fail to show up or cancel their scheduled appointments. These comments should be entered into the general quality-management data system for use in setting priorities for future continuity-of-care studies.

Medical Record Reviews

The patient's medical record contains important information that tells the health plan a lot about the continuity of that patient's health care. Clinical documentation in the record is essential in verifying continuity of care. Treatment may have been appropriate and timely; however, if the care rendered was not documented, this could lead to duplication of testing, overmedication, or inappropriate treatment and lack of continuity of care. This is particularly true when multiple physicians or disciplines are involved. In a health plan, the primary care provider (PCP) is the gatekeeper of care, and it is essential that he or she receives records documenting care provided outside of the office. If the health plan has regularly scheduled medical record reviews at its clinics, continuity-of-care questions can be added to the review criteria. For example, receipt of referral/consultation notes, laboratory tests, or ancillary services reports are matched against the request documented in the medical record, that is, the time of the order is compared with the date of receipt of information. See figure 9-3 for the kinds of information that can be evaluated during medical record reviews.

☐ Staffing Requirements

Once continuity-of-care quality indicators are defined by the health plan, identification of the departments or personnel responsible for data collection must be established. Data-gathering duties and referral to the QM department may be assigned to the staff members that have frequent and direct contact with members and providers, that is, claims examiners, medical record coders and abstractors, utilization review personnel, member services, or the marketing department personnel. Integration of utilization/quality management activities is essential in preventing duplication of the data-collection and report-generation processes. Staff involvement is key to ensuring their "buy-in" (acceptance or participation).

Evaluating the continuity of care at a health plan often requires the cooperation and involvement of the provider office staff. However, interference with work flow in the provider office must be minimized if a successful and meaningful evaluation is to be performed. The health plan's staffing requirements for collecting data about the quality of care continuity will vary according to the organization of the health plan and its internal data management resources. At a minimum, data collection and reporting will require an individual who has knowledge of automated systems and who can assist in identifying data elements and designing necessary reports. In larger plans, responsibility for report generation may involve various departments including claims, data analysis, and utilization review. However, the department assigned quality review and reporting responsibilities must have sufficient working knowledge of the entire health plan system in order to effectively communicate data needs to these other departments.

Some other variables to be considered in determining the number of health plan staff required for assessment and improvement activities include:

- The number of medical record reviews to be completed each year (frequency of ongoing studies and complexity of focused or special periodic studies).
- Where data collection will occur (labor costs for the health plan can be very expensive if many records in each clinic are reviewed rather than having clinic

Figure 9-3. Medical Record Review Criteria

1. Records contain consultation notes, laboratory tests, or ancillary services reports resulting from requests/orders noted in chart.

2. Emergency services records are maintained in the chart. (Emergency encounter information can be obtained from the claims data base prior to the medical record review visit and compared to the information located in the chart.)

3. Patient release of records to referred provider is annotated in the chart with documentation that the records were sent.

personnel collect and submit data items as part of their internal monitoring program).

- The availability of computerized support for data collection and reporting purposes.

☐ Reporting Quality-Review Results

Continuity-of-care reports are usually derived from several different sources within the organization, including grievance reports, referral/utilization patterns, claim/encounter data, and results of focused studies or medical record reviews.

To enable accurate analysis of the data, regardless of the source, trending of information is essential. This allows the health plan and its providers to look for patterns that may not be apparent in case-by-case analyses. A sample statistical report of quality measures related to continuity of care is shown in figure 9-4. This report provides an overview of the sources of continuity-of-care complaints and the types of quality problems identified for a full 12 months. The information for each calendar quarter is displayed, making it easier to identify patterns or trends needing investigation. The analysis, recommendations, and actions to be taken when patterns are identified are documented at the bottom of the report.

Other methods of reporting include the plan's provider newsletter, which could be used as the vehicle to inform the contracting network of quality assessment program results. The health plan's quality management staff should also communicate on a regular basis with the governing body, medical director, appropriate department heads, and health plan committees. A sample report for these groups is shown in figure 9-5. This more detailed report includes the specific results of studies and other review activities performed during a particular quarter and short narratives describing the issues that prompted investigation and action.

☐ Making Improvements

When a problem in continuity is identified, all appropriate health plan departments and representatives of the provider network should be involved in recommending and implementing necessary changes. For example, the contracting department may need to add contract language that addresses continuity-of-care issues if studies show that this addition will enhance providers' commitment to continuity.

Quality management of the continuity of care should include constant efforts to improve the referral process. For example, providers who leave the area or retire from practice should be sure their patients receive a referral to an alternative provider. Clinics and health plans alike should make every effort to make this transition as smooth as possible. Adding new providers to the referral base should also be constantly evaluated to ensure that continuity of care is not affected by future loss of providers or unavailability of care (because of surgery, vacations, illness, and other emergencies).

Future improvements in the continuity of care will result from data automation. Automated patient reminders about preventive care and follow-up appointments will reduce the number of "lost" patients. Patient reports that are communicated through modem or electronic mail (EM) to improve the timeliness of provider-to-provider communication will greatly enhance the continuity of care. These technologies will become more common in future years, and health plans must consider these new systems in their strategic planning related to continuity of care.

The ambulatory care organization may also consider becoming more involved in community health care, through immunization clinics, mammography screening programs, and other preventive programs delivered in the patients' neighborhoods.

119

Figure 9-4. Sample Statistical Report for Continuity-of-Care Quality Measurement

Date of Report and Analysis: 1/15/92

Continuity-of-Care Problems	Identified Through Surveys				Identified By Case Managers				Identified By Focused Studies			
	Jan.–Mar.	Apr.–June	July–Sept.	Oct.–Dec.	Jan.–Mar.	Apr.–June	July–Sept.	Oct.–Dec.	Jan.–Mar.	Apr.–June	July–Sept.	Oct.–Dec.
Access time for urgent care visit is not within plan standards	0	3	2	2	0	0	0	0	3	2	4	0
There is a lack of documentation of provider compliance with well-baby preventive care standards	0	0	0	0	1	0	0	0	4	2	0	0
Patients are receiving duplicate medication from different providers	0	1	0	0	0	4	0	1	0	0	0	3
Provider records lack notation of patient's medication allergies	0	0	0	0	0	0	1	0	0	0	0	12
Patients are missing scheduled appointments	0	0	0	0	2	0	2	4	0	1	0	1
There is a lack of documentation of patient education on preventive care	0	1	5	0	0	0	0	0	9	0	0	5

Analysis of Quality Report Findings

Problems in patient access for urgent-care appointments have been substantiated by patient survey and focused studies done in provider offices.

Three provider documentation issues have been identified: (1) well-baby preventive care, (2) patient allergies, and (3) patient education on preventive care.

Recommendations

Through focused study in January 1992, identify which provider specialty groups are delaying access for urgent care beyond 24 hours.

Update provider contracts to include reference to documentation requirements of health plan participation.

Actions

No further action will be taken until focused study is completed in January 1992.

Refer contract language change to medical director for inclusion in contract revision to be distributed in May 1992.

Figure 9-5. Quarterly Detail Report for the Medical Director, Department Heads, and Governing Board

July–Sept. 1991

Study/ Review Criteria	Study Population	Time Period	Number Failing Criteria	Medical Director Review	QA Committee Review	Quality Problems Identified
Specialist had patient information at time of referral visit	100 patient surveys	July 1991	5	5	3	1
No treatment delays were attributed to lack of information or test delays	100 patient surveys	July 1991	1	1	1	0
All recommended preventive education was discussed with patient	100 patient surveys	July 1991	23	23	23	10
Referrals were available to patients in a timely manner	20 provider surveys	July 1991	1	0	1	0
There were no providers to whom plan providers no longer refer patients	20 provider surveys	July 1991	0	0	0	0
Number of phone or written patient complaints regarding continuity	All plan members	July– Sept. 1991	2	2	2	0

Topic	Discussion	Action
QA committee identified one case in which a referral physician did not have information about a patient prior to a scheduled visit.	Reports of mammography findings were important for surgeon to review prior to patient visits for breast mass evaluation.	Letter was sent to primary care physician regarding slowness in communicating information to referral physician.
QA committee identified a trend regarding preventive health care education not being provided by primary care physicians.	Preventive health care education is important to patients' health status, and deficiency is important to correct.	News item was placed in October provider newsletter outlining preventive education recommendations. Plans were made to do medical record review at provider offices in January 1992 as follow-up to see if education and documentation of same have improved.
Prior authorization staff and case managers identified the need to add another nephrologist on provider plan because the one nephrologist on the panel was unable to manage the current patient load.	QA committee discussed with medical director its choices for other nephrologists.	Plans were made to solicit one more nephrologist by inviting those in the market area to apply for provider panel membership. Further discussion will occur after this solicitation in September 1991.

Continuity-of-care programs for certain disease processes—that is, AIDS, cancer, mental health, and geriatrics—will certainly become standard for specialty clinics.

☐ Conclusion

Patient and provider surveys, referral management protocols, specific contractual requirements, focused studies including review of encounter/paid claims data, medical record protocols/reviews, preventive care standards, and patient reminders are just a few examples of methods that managed care programs can implement to objectively measure and address continuity of care in an ambulatory care setting. If continuity of care is successfully attained, a health plan may enjoy a more efficient delivery system that will contain or reduce spiraling health care costs through effective preventive care, early diagnosis of diseases, prompt initiation of treatment, and ultimate reduction in patient morbidity. Ongoing evaluation and improvement in the continuity of patient health care services will ultimately improve the quality of care for health plan members. The documentation that comes out of this quality management program allows purchasers of health care to select the best value in quality health care.

☐ References

1. Office of Prepaid Health Care. *Quality Assurance Guidelines for Health Maintenance Organizations and Competitive Medical Plans.* Washington, DC: Health Care Financing Administration, 1986. 42 CRF 110.107 (c) (1).

2. Accreditation Association for Ambulatory Health Care, Inc. *Accreditation Handbook for Ambulatory Health Care.* 1990 Edition. Skokie, IL: AAAHC, 1989, p. 40.

3. American Cancer Society. Guidelines for cancer-related check-up: recommendations and rationale. *Cancer* 30:194–240, 1980.

4. American Cancer Society. Mammography, 1982: a statement of the ACS. *Cancer* 32:226–30, 1982.

5. National Cancer Institute. *Working Guidelines for Early Cancer Detection: Rationale and Supporting Evidence to Decrease Mortality.* Bethesda, MD: NCI, 1987.

6. McPhee, S. J., and Bird, J. A. Implementation of cancer prevention guidelines in clinical practice. *Journal of General Internal Medicine* 5(suppl):S116–S122, 1990.

7. U.S. Preventive Services Task Force. *Guide to Clinical Preventive Services.* Baltimore, MD: Williams & Wilkins, 1989.

Chapter 10

Continuity of Care among Hospital-Based Ambulatory Care Providers

---

Elizabeth C. Doherty, Ph.D.

Measuring the quality of continuity of care in the provision of ambulatory care services is a special challenge. While *continuity of care* implies the progression of a predetermined plan for health care services without disruption of the plan, *ambulation*, and thus ambulatory care, is defined as itinerant or moving from place to place. Hence the client of ambulatory care, unlike the hospitalized patient, is not as easily controlled, monitored, or guided through the health care processes. For this reason, the client of ambulatory care must be a more active player in the health care process if it is to be successful. This concern alone substantiates the need for close monitoring of continuity of care.

Traditional continuity-of-care quality monitors have included at a minimum (1) missed appointments that are not further reviewed or evaluated for trends; (2) scheduled laboratory tests or imaging procedures that never occur; (3) results of testing services that never find their way into the medical record or at least are not posted in a timely manner; and (4) lack of documentation of clinical findings in the medical record, including lack of signature and dating of the entry by the physician or other clinicians.[1] Three other quality monitors may also effectively evaluate continuity of care in the ambulatory care program, depending on the nature of the care required or offered and the setting of the program. These are monitors of (1) referral for consultation by a specialist without adequate documentation of clinical findings and test results, (2) referral for surgery or hospitalization without the aforementioned documentation, and (3) inadequate medical record documentation where there is a multiphysician staff rotation or where medical residents rotate through the ambulatory care program every several weeks.

☐ Continuity of Care at the University of Pittsburgh Medical Center

At the University of Pittsburgh Medical Center (UPMC), monitoring continuity of care in the ambulatory care environment includes the above-mentioned traditional monitors as well as specialized evaluations unique to each individual service. The UPMC offers a complex variety of ambulatory care services, with approximately 25 ambulatory care programs and services supported by or affiliated with the medical complex. These include three community health centers, each with multiple clinical programs; the Pittsburgh Cancer Institute; an HIV outpatient clinic; a pain center; two outpatient programs providing home care services; a durable medical equipment (DME) company, which deals primarily with in-home services; a maxillofacial program that qualifies as a DME because it creates facial and related prostheses; a sports medicine program; an outpatient physical therapy center; an ophthalmic laser center; a large emergency treatment department with several specialty areas; outpatient dental programs; a diabetes center; a dialysis center; speech and hearing programs; specialized vision services; and outpatient surgical services.

The uniqueness of a health care system this elaborate requires an expanded definition of the concept of continuity of care. In this particular system, evaluating continuity of care requires quality management systems that extend from the ambulatory/outpatient services to the inpatient environment, if necessary, and/or through additional ambulatory/outpatient services, including home care. A simple illustration of the continuity of care at UPMC is shown in figure 10-1.

The UPMC ambulatory care departments constantly monitor patient flow and communication about a patient's care in an effort to avoid customary interruptions in the continuity-of-care process. Ambulatory care departments evaluate waiting times between client arrival and initiation of treatment intervention or start of therapy. This quality monitor is common to several programs. Ambulatory care departments trend waiting time data to identify and eliminate events that cause clients to leave the site and perhaps never return. Several departments telephone clients the day before a scheduled appointment to remind them of the appointment, the day after treatment to inquire about treatment outcome, or both. Department staff may contact the patient the day after he or she has missed a scheduled appointment to ascertain why the appoint-

Figure 10-1. Continuity-of-Care Cycle for Ambulatory Care Services

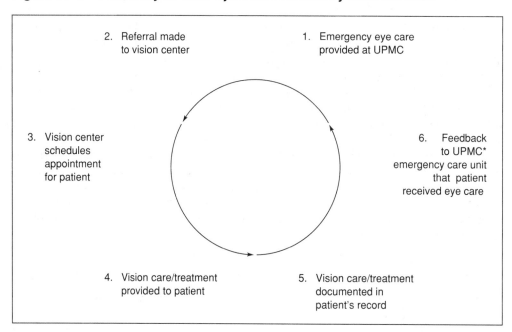

2. Referral made to vision center

1. Emergency eye care provided at UPMC

3. Vision center schedules appointment for patient

6. Feedback to UPMC* emergency care unit that patient received eye care

4. Vision care/treatment provided to patient

5. Vision care/treatment documented in patient's record

*UPMC = University of Pittsburgh Medical Center.

ment was not kept. The intent of this call is to arrange for rescheduling of the appointment.

Appropriateness of prescribed treatment or referrals for same and clinical pertinence of ordered tests are other quality measures used by many of the ambulatory care departments. The results of such monitors are trended to identify quality-of-care concerns as well as continuity-of-care problems. High on the quality evaluation list for all departments is the measurement of client satisfaction as an important aspect of continuity of care. If clients are not satisfied, they will most assuredly go elsewhere.[2] Although this topic is the subject of another chapter in this book, it must be noted that satisfaction with the care received, its timeliness, communication with the client throughout the ambulatory care experience, and the performance of the care givers are measures used by every ambulatory care department at UPMC.

☐ Quality Management Program Overview

Measures of the quality of health care continuity are researched, developed, and approved within each ambulatory care service throughout the UPMC system. Thresholds are likewise determined by each department: internal staff are deemed to be the most experienced in knowing what the expected outcomes ought to be. Data are generally collected by the individual staff of each department. However, each ambulatory care department has a representative of the facilities' Quality Improvement Department who serves as a liaison with the facilitywide quality management program. This contact or resource person assists the department with the development of quality monitors and at times assists with data collection or helps to identify additional sources of information for data retrieval. Such sources of information may include a number of computerized data bases within the medical center that contain information about all inpatients and outpatients seen by a particular service.

Standard references are used for developing quality monitors and for establishing thresholds or standards. These sources include the standards of the Joint Commission on Accreditation of Healthcare Organizations (JCAHO), the Pennsylvania Department of Health, the American Association of Blood Banks, the College of American Pathology, the American College of Surgeons' Commission on Cancer, the University Hospital Consortium, the National Institutes of Health, the Centers for Disease Control, and others. However, most important to the quality efforts are the day-to-day experiences of the staff who work with the clients in each ambulatory care program. Patient care experiences frequently yield unique yet meaningful quality concerns and help identify ways of collecting data to substantiate quality. For example, staff in the outpatient physical therapy department might notice that patients are arriving for their first appointment without copies of pertinent health history information from the primary care physician's office. By tallying the number of times this continuity-of-care problem occurs, which can easily be done by staff during the initial patient assessment, the quality problem can be substantiated and corrective action taken immediately. In addition, ambulatory care departments focus their quality review efforts on high-volume, high-risk, and problem-prone services and treatments.

Departments are encouraged to use both electronic and manual data-retrieval methods. Reliance on computer programs that claim to measure everything but inhibit the department's ability to adapt the software to its unique requirements is discouraged. Sophisticated spreadsheets and multiple overlapping graphs that demand road maps for interpretation are not a requirement for meaningful quality management at UPMC. Rather, PC-based information systems that allow the user to design simple forms and reports and can receive downloaded information from facilitywide mainframe data bases are more than satisfactory for every ambulatory care department. Even without hospital or large computer system backing for the ambulatory care department (as in the case of freestanding centers), programs designed with user-friendly software packages generate sufficient data to sustain a worthwhile ambulatory care quality management effort.

Once the quality data are collected and analyzed by the ambulatory care program staff, a report is presented first to the internal staff and then quarterly to the ambulatory care quality improvement committee (ACQIC). This committee, whose members include physicians providing ambulatory care services and management representatives from each of the ambulatory care departments, is charged with overseeing quality improvement activities in the entire ambulatory care division at UPMC. In addition to evaluating the adequacy of quality review activities performed at the department level, this committee works to ensure that each department's quality improvement focus is consistent with the goals of the ambulatory care division as a whole.

On a staggered schedule at each monthly ACQIC meeting, the ambulatory care departments summarize their quality review findings, actions, and progress in improving quality of care and service. Departments are encouraged to use two simple forms for reporting their quality review findings, recommendations, actions, and evaluations of the effectiveness of the actions taken. The quality of care/service report (figure 10-2) documents each of the quality measures being used by the department, and the results of data collection are entered each month. By presenting each month's results, the department and the ACQIC can identify trends that might not be apparent if only one month or one quarter of data were displayed. Each department documents the improvement projects it has undertaken on the monthly analysis of improvement activities (figure 10-3). The "Issue for Improvement" might include topics that were identified through regular quality indicator measures or through other sources (for example, patient complaints, staff recommendations, referrals from other departments). For each issue presented on the report, the department documents the recommendations/actions being taken to improve quality and the status of the improvement project. The ACQIC uses this report to track the progress of all identified improvement issues in each department and to ensure that corrective actions are being taken appropriately. The form in figure 10-3 may also be used for recording meeting minutes, with the first column heading changed to "Conclusions/Findings" for minute-taking purposes.

☐ Continuity-of-Care Quality Monitors for Specific Ambulatory Care Units

Use of the JCAHO's 10-step model for monitoring and evaluation[3] is the only requirement for the quality management programs in ambulatory care units at UPMC. Use of this model and a strong quality improvement commitment by individual program staff have resulted in successful programs. Many of the quality monitors of continuity of care described in chapter 9, such as inadequate medical record documentation, patient noncompliance, delays in treatment, and so forth, are used in UPMC's ambulatory care departments' quality management programs. In addition, departments focus on issues of particular importance to their unit and the clients they serve. A discussion of the quality monitors peculiar to individual departments follows.

Durable Medical Equipment Services

The durable medical equipment (DME) service provides in-home care and services including IV infusion therapy, oxygen therapy, and all types of medical equipment support (wheelchairs, walkers, hospital beds, and so forth). Its quality monitoring efforts focus on the quality of service provided and patient satisfaction. All new customers of

Figure 10-2. Example of Quality of Care Report (top) and Sample Report Form (bottom)

Department: Clinical Social Work Services							Date of Report: July 15, 1991						
Quality/Appropriateness Measures	**Threshold**	**Jan.**	**Feb.**	**Mar.**	**Apr.**	**May**	**June**	**July**	**Aug.**	**Sept.**	**Oct.**	**Nov.**	**Dec.**
Percentage of referred clients seen the day of referral	95%	85%	92%	98%	95%	98%	100%						
Percentage of records complete and appropriately documented	90%	82%	97%	91%	95%	100%	100%						
Percentage of clinical social workers in compliance with continuing education requirements	100%	100%	(1)	(1)	(1)	(1)	(1)						
Patient satisfaction with clinical social work services	95%	95%	NA	NA	93%	NA	NA						
Clients contacted by phone within 24 hours of missed appointment	98%	100%	100%	100%	91%	96%	100%						

Notes: This is an example of a reporting method. This is not an actual report from any hospital program.
(1) = Measure only reported quarterly or yearly.
NA = Data not available.

Quality of Care/Service Report

Department: _____ Date of Report: _____

Quality/Appropriateness Measures	Jan.	Feb.	Mar.	Apr.	May	June	July	Aug.	Sept.	Oct.	Nov.	Dec.

Figure 10-3. Monthly Analysis of Improvement Activities

Department: Clinical Social Work Services	Date of Report: July 15, 1991	
Issue for Improvement	**Recommendations/Actions**	**Status of Improvement Activities**
Low percentage of referred clients seen the day of referral during first quarter	A. Reorganized staff to provide better coverage over weekends.	Second-quarter results showed significant improvement.
Three written complaints were received from patients' families concerning service not received while visiting Emergency Department. Social workers were available at times noted in each complaint but were not requested by ED.	A. Attended Emergency Department Nursing Staff meeting 6/23/91. Discussed referral mechanisms for getting help for patients.	Continue to monitor for improved communication between departments.
Decline in number of patients reached by phone contact within 24 hours of missed appointment.	A. Corrected staffing shortage. Reminded all staff of the importance of this communication.	Problem resolved.

a DME service receive a satisfaction questionnaire with their first month's billing. The questionnaire, which was originally designed to evaluate the initial installation of the service or product, was revised to include questions measuring the customer's satisfaction with continuity-of-care issues. For example, was the equipment timely in arriving? Were instructions adequate? Was service unnecessarily interrupted for any reason? When questions arise after the initial installation, does the client receive timely and appropriate responses? Is there adequate medical intervention when the client's DME service needs change? Are the equipment vendors responsive to the medical and emotional needs of the client? Early identification of trends in these potentially problematic areas can reduce or eliminate continuity-of-care concerns.

Vision Center

The quality management program at the vision center evaluates overutilization and underutilization of resources by identifying clients who are unable or unwilling to participate in a particular treatment. To prevent disruption of services, vision center staff must identify these clients early in the treatment phase. If case review reveals that a client is not a candidate for a particular treatment plan, consideration is given for another mode of treatment to minimize interruptions or delays in health services. Experience in the vision center has shown that when clients perceive themselves as unable to cooperate with the prescribed treatment, they become discouraged and quietly withdraw from all further care. Early intervention is important to prevent a breakdown in the vision care delivery system.

Rehabilitation Services

Departments such as outpatient physical therapy and occupational therapy regularly monitor clients' utilization of services as a measure of continuity of care. Questions such as "What is an appropriate client/therapist ratio?" help to minimize problems with clients becoming discouraged and dropping out of therapy because of their perceived lack of attention from the therapist due to program overcrowding. Other questions that help identify continuity-of-care problems include:

- How long should therapy continue?
- How many treatments are required for the client to reach his or her maximum potential?
- How long will the therapy be covered by insurance?

These questions allow care givers to explore many aspects of the continuity-of-care issue.

Home Care Services

Like the contracted services of the DME and the vision center, the home care department evaluates overutilization and underutilization as a measure of continuity of care. Clients are accepted for home care only if needed services are available. Once the assessment for admission is completed, the determination for admission is announced. If the services needed for appropriate continuity of care are not available through the home care department, then an alternative care program must be found in order to ensure that care is uninterrupted.

Home care personnel visit their clients within 24 hours of receiving a referral. Evaluating compliance with this standard is a measure of continuity of care. The assessment for admission to home care is conducted and the plan of care develops from this step forward. The medical necessity of home care for each client must be recertified for insurance purposes at least every 60 days. If necessary, the client's care plan is revised to reflect the progressive care needs of the client and to document the need for continuation of home care services. Regular monitoring of the care plan documentation is conducted by the department director to ensure that services are continued only when medically appropriate. Further in-depth review of the entire home care record occurs quarterly and more often if an unannounced visit from the department of health occurs.

Maxillofacial Prosthesis Department

Continuity of care is extremely important both as a clinical concept and as a quality monitor for clients of the Maxillofacial Prosthetics Department. In many cases, the client has undergone surgery for cancer, birth defects, or trauma repair prior to referral to this outpatient service. The measure of continuity of care becomes more obvious and perhaps more formal here, as with home care, in that a discharge plan has been initiated for these clients prior to their release from the hospital. The maxillofacial prosthesis staff design and create their own product line for their ambulatory care population. This service enhances clients' quality of life by providing prostheses to damaged areas of the head and neck. Quality monitoring centers on the acceptance or rejection of the prosthesis by the client. The quality of the prosthesis itself is very important because of its effect on the client's acceptance of this seemingly drastic adaptation in life. Clients' acceptance of their prostheses is regularly evaluated, with the threshold for acceptance set at slightly under 100 percent.

The maxillofacial prothesis service is considered a DME service because it creates its own appliances for client rehabilitation. Hence insurance coverage issues are also a part of this department's quality management program. A high rate of insurance coverage denials can affect the continuity of care if the client's personal financial resources are insufficient.

Oncology and Speech Therapy Departments

The ambulatory care departments of oncology and speech therapy evaluate continuity of care by monitoring client treatment goals—whether the care plan is completed and to what extent accomplishment of goals is realistic. These two ambulatory care services generally are used after a client's inpatient surgery or treatment for primary tumors. A comprehensive continuing care plan is documented for these clients through the hospital's discharge-planning process. To ensure continuity, the oncology and speech therapy staff constantly evaluate the efficiency of communication between the inpatient provider and their outpatient counterparts. There are times when interruptions in the treatment process are unavoidable. However, each case is reviewed independently with the department's quality standards in mind. Staff of these two ambulatory care areas are sensitive to the client's clinical and emotional needs. Through early identification of treatment interference problems, the staff can encourage the client to keep returning for care until the designated plan of treatment is completed.

In these two ambulatory care areas an important measure of quality is staff performance, which is viewed as a pivotal aspect of continuity of care that can contribute to or inhibit the client from continuing treatment. Client–staff communication is vital to the continuity of care because the client must perceive that he or she is getting enough attention or assistance. Furthermore, clients must know what their responsibilities are in the treatment process. Is the treatment active or passive? Do they need constant supervision, or can they continue the treatment with minimal help, once instructed? If these matters are not addressed proactively, continuity of care and health care problem resolution can be adversely affected.

Outpatient Laboratory Services

Outpatient laboratories play a vital role in preserving continuity of care. Laboratory professionals know how essential their services are to clients at UPMC ambulatory care departments. For example, clients receiving chemotherapy at the Pittsburgh Cancer Institute or those receiving radiation treatments at the ambulatory oncology service can be adversely affected by poor-quality laboratory services. The length of client waiting time between blood being drawn and test results being reported back to the respective center is an important quality measure for the laboratory. Results must be available before treatment can begin to ensure that doses of chemotherapy or radiation are accurate for the client's needs. The outpatient laboratory services set standards and measure compliance with the timeliness of blood sampling procedures and reporting accuracy and efficiency. Knowing these parameters of care contributes to minimizing the client's time spent at the facility and thus improves satisfaction with services. The outpatient laboratory services monitor the following:

- Patient waiting time
- Time needed to complete a phlebotomy
- Transport time of the sample
- "Stat" and routine test turnaround times

Additionally, the outpatient laboratories evaluate the quality of the specimen collection process through periodic assessments of the behavior of collection personnel, compliance with patient identification procedures, appropriateness of specimen choice in relation to the test ordered, and specimen rejection rates. Each of these quality measures provides important data about the laboratory performance and helps identify issues that can affect continuity of care.

Clinical Social Work Services

Clinical social work services provide the most important link between the ambulatory care and inpatient providers and the health care clients. There would be many more breakdowns in the continuity of care without the social workers' constant attention to detail and their assistance with finding available and appropriate services, helping the client with financial issues, arranging transportation for the client to the ambulatory care program, and many more enabling tasks. For the hospitalized patient nearing the end of his or her stay, clinical social workers implement the discharge plan by contacting ambulatory care services for assessment of the client's needs, initiating posthospital services, or both. For the ambulatory care client, whether hospitalization has occurred or not, social workers provide the link from one service to another. Equally important, they provide the shoulder to lean on and the encouragement to continue the care process until the treatment is concluded or the problem is resolved as effectively as possible.

At UPMC, clinical social work services are the communication link between the client and the clinic's care givers. In addition to coordinating clinical services, social workers assist clients with resolving personal or emotional problems that influence the client's participation in the clinical care. It is important that these matters be well documented so that the care givers understand what environmental influences the client is coping with while simultaneously undergoing medical care. What is all-important, then, is the thoroughness and conciseness of the clinical social workers' documentation in the client's medical or home care record. Many of the quality measures of clinical social work services focus on the completeness of record documentation.

Through periodic questionnaires that collect clients' perceptions of staff performance, the Clinical Social Work Department makes constant improvements in its quality of care. Included in these surveys are questions assessing the clinical social workers' capacity to express sincere sympathy and empathy, the timeliness of their services, the clarity with which they communicate the discharge plan of care, and how well the plan of care meets the client's needs and wishes. Other ongoing monitors of the quality of clinical social work services in relation to continuity of care include:

- Percentage of referred clients seen the day of referral
- Percentage of clients' medical records that document initial social work assessment or ongoing visits according to department standards within 48 hours of the initial visit
- Number of clients who miss two consecutive medical specialty clinic visits and how actively they are contacted and encouraged to resume care
- Completeness and appropriateness of the documentation in the medical record
- Quality of the medical center coach service that transports patients who may be two to four hours away or who are coming from the airport to the UPMC programs
- Timeliness of responses to requests for temporary housing needs for out-of-town clients who need to continue with the ambulatory care program for a few days or weeks
- Effectiveness of client interviewing basic to the provision of fundamental housing and living needs
- Efficiency in closing of cases that are no longer active

Another important continuity-of-care measure is the identification of clients who are referred for clinical social work consultation but who do not wait to see the clinical social worker. Social workers evaluate the reasons why clients insist they could not stay, especially for the first referral visit, by telephoning the client within 24 hours of the missed appointment. Clinical social work services look for chronic problems such as transportation needs or inappropriate appointment scheduling as reasons for missed appointments.

Whereas the medical record is frequently the source of data on quality for ambulatory care, including clinical social work services, staff must remember that the measure of quality focuses on aspects of patient care even though the data are obtained from the medical record. For example, the clinical social work services originally had defined one of their quality indicators as "percentage of medical records reviewed that contained an appropriate psychosocial assessment, as defined by the department policy, within 48 hours of receipt of the consultation request." To spotlight the clinical component being measured, the indicator was changed to "percentage of patients receiving appropriate psychosocial assessment within 48 hours of receipt of the consultation request." Although both indicators measured the same aspect of care, the wording of the new indicator emphasized the patient rather than the documentation viewpoint.

The Medical Record

Just as clinical social work is considered an important communication link between the medical care givers and the clients of ambulatory care, of equal importance as a communication link are the medical record and the quality and completeness of the information contained in it. The medical record is the instrument of communication that guides the continuity of care efficiently, effectively, and with high-quality performance. Reports and documentation of all planning and assessments, all treatment and interventions, and the client's health care outcome come together in this one central location. Medical record review is an ongoing, multidisciplinary activity in all ambulatory care departments. Because of this somewhat loosely structured ambulatory care atmosphere, it is much easier to lose track of what services were rendered, what plans were made, and in general what happened to the client along the way.

Ambulatory care departments at UPMC conduct frequent record reviews as a starting point for additional quality evaluations. Findings from record review tell as much about how the client is progressing as they do about the quality of the contents of the record. If documentation is complete, accurate, and appropriate, then continuity of care for all clients becomes a more realistic goal. Staff rotations become somewhat less hazardous, and the continued care of the client becomes more effective when all of the documentation is in place.

☐ Effectiveness of the Quality Management Program

Through the quality management process in the UPMC ambulatory care departments, services that rely on each other to "close the loop" or eliminate delays and interruptions in treatment have become more conscious of the interdependence they share in the continuity of care for each client. As a result of monitoring turnaround service times, timeliness of response, waiting times, and similar quality indicators, ambulatory care departments have made great strides toward improving the timeliness and appropriateness of testing, records, and patient directions and instructions (to mention a few).

Knowing that they will eventually share their quality monitoring results with others, ambulatory care department staff go to great lengths to make sure the data are accurately represented and well displayed. As the quality improvement and legal departments make confidentiality of information a key point, practitioners appear to communicate more effectively, reassured that the information discussed will assist others in doing a better, more efficient job without practitioners worrying about information leaks. Materials presented at meetings are collected and destroyed at the conclusion of the meetings. Official records are kept in the department office and in the quality assurance office. These confidentiality procedures are important to freestanding ambulatory care centers as well as community service agencies. Files should have locks and shredding machines should be readily available.

☐ Conclusion

A quality management program like the one at UPMC can work only if there is visible and proactive support from the governing body, administration, and the medical staff.

Ambulatory care service providers must commit to quality with the realization that quality management activities are an integral part of their day-to-day responsibility to ensure continuity of care for each and every client. Even if only one of the links in this chain is weak, the health care system will not work to capacity. The various departments and staff must not be afraid to take a risk or make suggestions. Individual creativity is important in pulling the service or program effort together. Resources are available; they need not be expensive or complicated. Simple and concise methods will afford an effective and efficient quality management program for all ambulatory care providers.

☐ References

1. Joint Commission on Accreditation of Healthcare Organizations. *Quality Assurance in Ambulatory Care.* 2nd ed. Chicago: JCAHO, 1990, p. 50.

2. Weiss, B. D., and Senf, J. H. Patient satisfaction survey instrument for use in health maintenance organizations. *Medical Care* 28(5):434–44, May 1990.

3. Joint Commission on Accreditation of Healthcare Organizations. *Monitoring and Evaluation: Physical Rehabilitation Services.* Chicago: JCAHO, 1988, pp. 17–24.

Section Six

Access to Health Care Services

To be successful, ambulatory care services must be available and accessible to patients with respect to geographic location, hours of operation, and provisions for after-hours services. Ambulatory care providers must ensure that services are not delayed or denied to patients. Evaluating patient access to health care services incorporates such factors as the empathetic art of caring that providers impart to their patients and the perceptions of the patient as to the quality of the product. Chapter 11 details patient and practitioner surveys, reviews of emergency department and hospital admissions, assessments of waiting time for appointments, and other techniques for ambulatory care providers to use in measuring the quality of patient care access.

Chapter 11

Measurement of Patient Access to Ambulatory Care

Pam Blackmore

Accessible health care can be defined as the ability of patients to receive health care services when medically necessary and with reasonable promptness. The evaluation of accessibility is a required quality management component for all federally certified health maintenance organizations (HMOs) and competitive medical plans. The Public Health Service Act provides broad authority for the federal government's quality assurance regulations. These regulations require HMOs and competitive medical plans to ensure that health care services are "available and accessible to members with reasonable promptness with respect to geographic location, hours of operation, and provisions for after-hours services. Medically necessary emergency services must be available 24 hours a day, 7 days a week."[1] Whether quality management is being performed by a health plan or the ambulatory care clinic itself, there are several methods for evaluating the quality of health care access.

Accessibility of care can be evaluated through the use of patient surveys, quality indicators, geographic patient/provider ratios, in-office waiting times, and appointment waiting times. This chapter describes quality management strategies related to accessibility for ambulatory care clinics, HMOs, individual practice associations (IPAs), and preferred provider organizations (PPOs).

☐ Establishing the Appraisal System

Measures of health care access vary according to the ambulatory health care delivery system being evaluated. Primary and specialty medical clinics, IPAs, HMOs, and PPOs will establish their evaluation systems to cover a myriad of services. Outpatient surgery clinics, radiology, and laboratory settings will focus their assessment activities on the specific services they provide. A variety of information sources can be used to identify health care access concerns. For example, a review of reports identifying problem-prone, high-risk, high-volume services is one way of determining areas that should be evaluated for accessibility of care. In many ambulatory health care environments, billing/encounter information is maintained in a computerized data base and can be used to target areas for a specialized review of health care access. Patient and provider complaints and grievances are another key source of information. Patient satisfaction surveys can also provide data that help in the measurement of health care accessibility. Health plans may find their risk management reports and litigation claims data to be valuable sources of identifying potential access problems. Finally, clinics or health plans with a formal quality management program already in place may turn to their existing measures of quality to identify trends that signal an accessibility concern.

Examples of common measures of health care accessibility include:

- Delays in treatment or diagnosis resulting in adverse outcome
- Waiting time for appointments (primary and specialty care):
  —Emergent appointment (not immediately available)
  —Urgent appointment (more than one day)
  —Routine appointment (more than six weeks)
- Waiting time for elective surgery exceeds "X" months
- Percentage of patients with scheduled appointments who wait more than "X" minutes in the clinic prior to being seen
- On-call telephone availability of staff within a given time period:
  —Calls for urgent problems are not returned within "X" minutes
  —Calls for nonurgent problems are not returned within "X" minutes
- Availability of after-hours care
- Number of patient complaints related to accessibility
  —Waiting time on hold
  —Number of hang ups for patient on hold

☐ Getting Approval of the Quality Measures

Approval of the quality indicators to be used for measuring accessibility of health care is important to ensure provider "buy-in" to the quality management program. If the quality review activities are being performed by an individual clinic, approval may be obtained from the physicians practicing at the clinic who may be on the clinic QM/Peer Review Committee.

Health plan program approval is the responsibility of the governing body. Some regionalized health plans do not have a local board of directors and must use an administrative committee to review and approve the quality measurement program. The health plan's medical director must be involved in the development of the quality measurements and the approval process. The provider community should be involved through representation on a health plan quality management committee. And, because day-to-day responsibilities for data-collection fall to the health plan's quality management staff, their input is important. Legal review is always helpful when establishing program requirements for accessibility of care. The health plan's lawyer is an excellent resource for interpreting regulatory requirements and evaluating the legal risk of poor patient care outcomes related to accessibility of care.

☐ Determining Thresholds

The Joint Commission on Accreditation of Healthcare Organizations (JCAHO), a forerunner in the development of quality indicators, points out that "the data collected for each (quality) indicator cannot alone lead to conclusions about the quality or appropriateness of care. Before collecting data, staff should agree on a threshold—an established level or point in the cumulative data that will trigger intensive evaluation. The threshold indicates that beyond this number or percentage, the staff is committed to looking into what could be a problem."[2] Thresholds for quality indicators that measure accessibility of care should be realistic. If the clinic or health plan has no experience in setting thresholds or defining standards of care, it is advisable to seek assistance from trade associations, professional societies, regulatory agencies, clinic/plan historical data, and current medical literature. Examples of thresholds, or minimal levels of quality as they relate to measuring health care access, are discussed in the following section.

Out-of-Plan Referrals

Counting "out-of-plan referrals" is one way that health plans evaluate accessibility. In California, HMOs use their state regulations as a basis for evaluating access to care through the percentage of services referred to noncontracting providers. In excess of 10 percent of total health care services provided by noncontracting providers is a signal that the provider network should be increased (State of California, Title 10, Section 1377).

Waiting Times

Different authors recommend different thresholds for patient waiting times in the clinic. Leland R. Kaiser, principal consultant for Kaiser and Associates, suggests that "when waiting time is longer than treatment time, patient dissatisfaction is compounded."[3] In the absence of historical data about clinic waiting times, consider setting a threshold between 20 and 30 minutes. This suggested waiting time is not the result of a formalized published study but instead is based on what seems to be reasonable and acceptable for patients waiting to see their physician. This is an average and would allow a range of shorter and longer times. Because unforeseen incidents can occur over which the provider has no control, that is, emergencies and hospital admissions, both the average waiting time and number of cases of excessive waiting time should be counted and reported.

Referral Waiting Times

Accessibility of health care can be measured by evaluating referral waiting times for appointments for emergent, urgent, and routine care for primary and specialty providers. Again, without historical data, thresholds may need to be arbitrarily set. Experience by clinics and health plans using this measure of health care access suggests that indicator thresholds also should be categorized into emergent, urgent, and routine appointments (or similar designations). An average waiting time combining these three types of appointments is not recommended. Definitions and thresholds for each of the appointment categories must be approved (see figure 11-1 for an example from one health plan's accessibility study).

Emergent Care

Patient access to medically necessary emergent care should be immediately available. If a clinic appointment is not possible or office care is not appropriate for the emergency, the patient should be referred to an emergency services facility *immediately*. The threshold for availability of emergency care may be either 0 percent or 100 percent—that is, in either case, even one occurrence of delayed emergency care would trigger a focused evaluation.

Urgent Care

Urgent appointments should be available within 24 hours. If the request for care is made late in the day, the clinic should refer the patient to an emergency or urgent care facility if a clinic appointment is not available. Again, the threshold for this measure of accessibility is 0 percent or 100 percent.

139

Figure 11-1. Patient Access to Physician Services: Definitions and Thresholds

Physical Examination: Patient with no health problem wishing a physical or with a chronic health problem.

Standard: Within 30 working days (six weeks).

First Referral Consultation: This is a non-urgent referral.

Standard: Within 10 working days (two weeks).

Routine Visits: These are routine follow-up examinations, routine pap smears, well-baby checks, and so forth.

Standard: Within 10 working days (two weeks).

Non-Urgent Visits: Conditions that require a visit. While not considered urgent, patients need to be seen in a timely fashion.

Standard: Within 5 working days (one week).

Urgent: Conditions that require medical intervention on the same day.

Standard: Same-day appointment.

Emergent: Conditions that require immediate medical intervention.

Standard: Within 30 minutes of notification of emergent situation.

Source: Reprinted, with permission, from Spath, P. (ed.). Access to quality: a quality monitor for ambulatory services. In: *Health Care Quality Assurance: Management and Methodologies.* Chicago: American Medical Record Association, Quality Assurance Section, 1990, p. 59.

Routine Care

The threshold for availability of routine care appointments will vary significantly according to provider. In most instances, routine care appointments should be available *within two to six weeks,* depending on the types of appointments (that is, routine visits, complete physical examinations, and preventive visits).

Some subspecialist appointments require longer waits because of their patient load and shortage of similar physician/providers of care in the immediate area. If the patient's health plan controls access to certain specialties, the health plan has a responsibility to contract with additional providers or the clinic must establish alternative referral patterns when a prolonged waiting period would jeopardize the patient's health.

Elective Surgery

Waiting times for elective surgery should be reasonable; a suggested threshold or waiting period is "not greater than three months." This threshold may vary according to the season: experience has shown the volume of surgery does vary throughout the year.

Office Care Availability

Primary care health care services need to be available 24 hours a day. For continuity of care and availability purposes, it is not advisable for the provider to sign out to the emergency room, or be without provision for an on-call replacement (with the same qualifications as the provider). Office hours should also be evaluated to determine whether the times are convenient for the clinic's or health plan's patient population. Regular office hours must be established because sporadic hours may reduce access to care by making it difficult for patients to schedule appointments. Because more adults in households are employed during weekday hours, availability of health care services after regular working hours and on weekends becomes even more important. Thresholds for quality indicators measuring health care availability should be set at reasonable levels, based on input from clinic physicians and all health plan providers.

Geographic Location

Clinic physicians should consider geographic access when referring patients for specialty, surgical, or ancillary services. If travel time or convenience is a concern to the patient, referrals may not be fulfilled and the quality of care may be compromised. Health plans have an obligation to ensure geographic access for their members, making this an important component of their measure of accessibility.[4] The contracting process of the health plan must include a review of the geographic location of network providers. The state of California HMO regulations require that the health plan provide access to care within a 15-mile radius or 30-minute travel time for their rural members. It is expected that these requirements will be exceeded for metropolitan areas [State of California, Title 10, Section 1300.51 (d)(H)(i)(ii)].

Case Load

Patients must be assured of sufficient time with their health care provider to allow for an accurate assessment of their health problem. Providers should establish a maximum patient load and compare this threshold to their current reality in order to confirm that their patient load is not excessive and individual patients are given the time they require. The provider must be able to determine the average number of patients he or she can adequately manage per hour. Some family practice providers are comfortable seeing four to six patients per hour, whereas some subspecialists may wish to see only two to four patients per hour. The number of patients who can be seen will vary by specialty type or patient mix (that is, elderly patients, patients with mental disorders, and so forth). Providers must also assess their ability to accept new patients versus maintaining their existing patient load.

To measure this aspect of accessibility, the provider's appointment book can be periodically evaluated to determine the number of patients seen per hour. These results are compared with the threshold to determine whether the averages appear to be excessive for the provider's specialty.

Patient/Provider Ratios

Patient/provider ratios can be calculated and reported as a way of identifying potential access problems. Patient/provider ratios are the number of patients who expect to receive health care service from an individual or group of providers. To ensure accessibility to necessary health care services, the clinic or health plan must determine whether it is possible for the physician or clinic to adequately service the number of patients linked to the provider and still maintain desired quality. Therefore, information such as the total number of patients affiliated with the provider is critical information.

Clinics and health plans must review individual patient/provider ratios on a regular basis to determine when additional providers must be added. In setting thresholds for this ratio, the state of California HMO regulations might be helpful. These standards require one FTE primary care provider for every 2,000 members and one FTE (primary and/or specialty provider) for every 1,200 members [State of California, Title 10, Section 1300.76.2(d)].

Determining full-time equivalency for a network HMO made up of providers who provide services to a multitude of health plans and payers can be difficult. One way to determine FTE needs for providers who deal with multiple payers is to determine the number of patients linked to the provider (regardless of payer source). Although there are no definitive methods for establishing a threshold when there are so many variables

141

to consider, it is possible to track the individual provider and monitor changes in the number of patients linked to the provider, complaints and grievances related to accessibility, number of patients seen per day, and office hours.

Language Requirements

The clinic or health plan must consider the language requirements of their patients or health plan members. The health care information must be accessible, meaning patients must be able to understand explanations and instructions about their health care. Clinic staff, printed information, telephone exchange personnel, and other individuals and documents should be readily available for the patient who does not speak English. This can be especially important for health plans that are responsible for maintaining information on their providers, including languages spoken. When patients express specific language needs, the clinic/health plan should be able to refer them to an appropriate provider.

☐ Collecting the Data

Once the clinic or health plan has identified ways of evaluating accessibility of care, the staff-assigned data-collection responsibilities must be identified. Data-collection may be delegated to health plan claims examiners, medical record specialists, utilization review personnel, member services or marketing department staff, clinic office staff, or quality management professionals.

In a health plan, as well as in the private clinic, all employees and providers should be encouraged to report concerns about health care access. However, primary data-collection responsibility for specific measures of accessibility should be assigned to those personnel who have frequent and direct contact with members and providers or have existing data-collection responsibilities (such as utilization review/quality management personnel in the health plan or medical record specialists in a clinic). Minimizing duplicative data-collection is essential to any quality measurement effort. This coordination is especially important in the evaluation of health care accessibility because these measures of quality may overlap with those used for other quality review purposes. By combining data-collection efforts and sorting the results into different reporting categories, that is, outcome, accessibility, continuity, and so forth, multiple aspects of ambulatory care quality can be assessed with only a few indicators of quality and with only minimal staff involvement.

A cost–benefit analysis is useful in selecting among different data-collection alternatives. Although 100 percent review of all cases is the most thorough method of reviewing accessibility of care, this type of analysis may increase the cost of health care because the costs may be prohibitive. Accessibility, although an important consideration in improving quality of care, requires the specific review of certain unique types of services. These special studies or program components must be considered in the budgetary process to ensure that adequate funds are available to successfully implement the anticipated program requirements. This requires the use of historical data to identify computer programming costs, personnel costs, mailing costs, and other expenses.

It is absolutely essential that data-collection tools and methods be developed prior to quality assessment implementation. During the planning stages it is also advisable that the data-collection tools be tested using actual medical or chart information to answer certain questions:

1. Is the information available?
2. What essential information is missing and what should be added?
3. Does the data-collection format impede the collection process?

4. Can the data be analyzed and presented in a simple, useful, and acceptable manner?
5. Are uniform reporting and data validation mechanisms included in the process?
6. Will the mere fact of collecting data cause variations in practices during the duration of the review effort? (Hawthorne effect)

A planned systematic process is necessary to collect and report preestablished quality measures efficiently. Data should be collected and referred to the quality management staff for evaluation, analysis, and reporting to various departments including providers, member/consumer services, utilization review, medical records, marketing, and claims/encounter or billing departments. Several different data sources are useful for collecting health care access information; these include surveys, encounter/billing information, complaints and grievances, case reviews, and medical records.

Provider/Patient Surveys

Questionnaires are useful on an ongoing basis for evaluating the effectiveness of the health care delivery system. Sample sizes that are large enough to provide statistically significant results must be used so that accurate conclusions can be drawn to assist in improving services. Surveys evaluating quality of care, including access, should be conducted at least annually. Specific questions related to accessibility can be incorporated into general satisfaction/quality surveys. Potential problem areas identified through the survey process will prompt more detailed analysis, that is, provider and member telephone interviews, one-on-one patient interviews, or written questionnaires.

Health plans that serve geographically different areas should release surveys that allow for results reported by region; this is done by color-coding the surveys. This can assist in recognizing accessibility-of-care issues that may be present only in certain regions. Sample accessibility questions for a health plan survey of patient satisfaction are shown in figure 11-2. Sample questions for a provider survey are shown in figure 11-3. These surveys are intended to be part of a larger study, with the questions shown in the figures addressing only accessibility issues. Demographic information including age, sex, and ambulatory care organization information should also be included on the survey, as well as space for comments and a phone number or address where individuals may contact the organization directly for comments or complaints, or to express satisfaction.

More internal staff may be needed to conduct surveys during the development phase, but they will not be needed when the same survey is repeated. Identification of the survey mailing list requires computerized reports or manual logs. Staffing requirements increase when manual processes are used to select survey participants for large patient populations. Staffing requirements will also change if the investigation is conducted by an independent survey firm. There are certain advantages to using an independent firm to develop and evaluate the surveys. An independent company can provide a more unbiased review and analysis of the results. This is particularly important when the results are used for marketing efforts or for complying with regulatory requirements.

Appointment waiting times can be evaluated by surveying the provider's appointment log through on-site review or written or telephone contacts. The clinic or health plan staff could call providers nights, weekends, and holidays to determine their availability. A data-collection form for documenting the results of appointment access is shown in figure 11-4 (p. 146).

Encounter/Billing Information

Encounter/billing information is another source for determining whether patients have appropriately accessed the health care system. For example, patients may not have

Figure 11-2. Patient Access Questions

---

1. The last time you saw your physician, were you able to schedule a routine office visit (that is, physical examination or preventive appointment) within (circle answer):

   a. 2 weeks
   b. 4 weeks
   c. 6 weeks
   d. Over 6 weeks

2. At your most recent clinic visit to see your primary physician, how long was the waiting period (time you arrived until you saw the physician) when you were in the office? (circle answer):

   a. 15 minutes or less
   b. 15 to 30 minutes
   c. 30 to 60 minutes
   d. 60 minutes or longer

3. The last time you saw a specialist, how long was the waiting period (time you arrived until you saw the specialist) when you were in the office? (circle answer):

   a. 15 minutes or less
   b. 15 to 30 minutes
   c. 30 to 60 minutes
   d. 60 minutes or longer
   e. I have never seen a specialist

5. Have you ever received emergency care?

   Yes _____   No _____

6. If "yes" to #5: Were you able to access this care immediately?

   Yes _____   No _____

7. Have you ever received urgent care? (This is for conditions not considered life-threatening but requiring care within the same day; may include care in the physicians' office or emergency room or clinic.)

   Yes _____   No _____

8. If "yes" to #7: Were you able to access this care within 24 hours?

   Yes _____   No _____

---

received immunizations according to organizational preventive care guidelines. Whereas this variation may represent a quality-of-care concern, the provider should also investigate the possibility of accessibility problems through a follow-up patient survey. Several questions related to infant immunizations may be included in this survey, such as:

1. Are both parents employed full-time?
2. Have the provider/clinic hours prevented the parents from scheduling the infant's well-baby appointments?
3. Are the insurance copayments too high or deductibles too restrictive, causing a decrease in the number of visits?

Encounter information may also be used to calculate the number of patients seen by the provider on a given day or an average number of patients seen per day. This number is useful in calculating provider caseloads. Referral management and utilization review data bases also provide an excellent source of information. Frequently, this information is more timely than claims/encounter data.

Complaints and Grievances

It is assumed that complaints and grievances are collected by the provider, clinic, or health plan. If patients confide that they were unable to make an appointment or waited

Figure 11-3. Provider Access Questions

1. Were other providers able to accept your referral patients within the following time frames:

   a. Emergent—Immediate

   Yes _____   No _____

   b. Urgent—Same day

   Yes _____   No _____

   c. Routine—4 to 6 weeks

   Yes _____   No _____

2. Are the following ancillary services available to your patients in a timely manner?

   a. Laboratory

   Yes _____   No _____

   b. Routine Radiology

   Yes _____   No _____

   c. Specialized Radiology

   Yes _____   No _____

   d. Durable Medical Equipment

   Yes _____   No _____

   d. Home Health

   Yes _____   No _____

3. Optional: If "no" to any of the above sections, please explain:

for one hour and left without seeing the provider, appropriate access to health care services was not attained. When the patient makes a verbal or written complaint, it is necessary to capture and trend this information to determine whether there is a pattern or continual problem within the health care delivery system. The clinic or health plan must have a system in place to make it easy for member/providers to complain: phone-line recorded message, an office within the clinic or health plan to allow for patients who walk in with complaints, or forms that are sent to patients during the enrollment process or provided during the actual clinic encounter. Clinic or health plan staff experiences and complaints are another source of information useful in identifying accessibility issues.

The number of complaints and grievances per 1,000 encounters or patients is one measure of quality and can be used to compare current-year experience with prior-year results. Grievances related to accessibility of care should be reported separately, allowing analysis of trends that require investigation. Separate reporting of complaints and grievances also provides follow-up data to evaluate the results of actions taken to improve accessibility.

Case Reviews

Quality-of-care and risk-management case reviews can also provide information on accessibility, particularly if the results of these reviews are tallied in such a way as to identify accessibility problems. Information obtained through case reviews can help providers and health plans unearth access problems. Data can be collected by all departments or individuals who have direct contact with patients/members. This in-

Figure 11-4.   Accessibility Evaluation Form

Medical Group: _____
Physician: _____
Date/Time of Review: _____

Routine Visit
Number of days between call and
available appointment:

_____ days

If physician was unable to see patient within
10 working days, record referral provider:

Visit Offered With:
_____ Physician requested
_____ Same clinic, another
            physician
_____ Physician requested,
            another clinic
_____ Another medical group
_____ Other: _____

Physical Examination
Number of days between call and
available appointment:

_____ days

If physician was unable to see patient
within 30 working days, record referral
provider:

Visit Offered With:
_____ Physician requested
_____ Same clinic, another
            physician
_____ Physician requested,
            another clinic
_____ Another medical group
_____ Other: _____

Non-Urgent
Number of days between call and
available appointment:

_____ days

If physician was unable to see patient
within 5 working days, record referral
provider:

Visit Offered With:
_____ Physician requested
_____ Same clinic, another
            physician
_____ Physician requested,
            another clinic
_____ Hospital emergency room
_____ Another medical group
_____ Other: _____

Urgent
Number of hours between call and
available appointment:

_____ hours

If physician was unable to see patient
within 1 day, record referral
provider:

Visit Offered With:
_____ Physician requested
_____ Same clinic, another
            physician
_____ Physician requested,
            another clinic
_____ Hospital emergency room
_____ Another medical group
_____ Other: _____

cludes the receptionist, nurses, and other providers in the clinic, as well as marketing, utilization review, and provider relations or consumer/member services departments in the health plan.

Medical Record Reviews

Medical record reviews are another avenue of information concerning accessibility of health care services. Figure 11-5 shows accessibility review criteria that can be included in the medical record review process. Medical record reviews may be conducted on an ongoing basis or periodically (quarterly). Because medical record reviews are time-consuming, it is important to integrate all data-collection activities with the record review process. For example, if continuity, accessibility, preventive care, and other quality management program studies require medical record reviews, these activities/ visits should be coordinated as much as possible to minimize interruption of providers and clinic staff and reduce duplication of data-collection efforts. This is most important

Figure 11-5. Medical Record Accessibility Review Criteria

---

1. Are appointments to referred providers accessed within the time periods established for the type of referral (emergent, urgent, and routine)?

   Yes _____   No _____   Not Applicable _____

2. Does the review of emergency records demonstrate accessibility of care necessary to treat condition?

   Yes _____   No _____   Not Applicable _____

3. Has the provider documented any problems in accessing needed treatment or diagnostic testing?

   Yes _____   No _____   Not Applicable _____

---

when health plan reviewers must schedule visits to independent offices. Providers are very careful with their staff resources and are not appreciative when seemingly unnecessary, repeated site visits occur.

□ Reporting Results

The data collected during the review process must be reported in such a way as to allow for analysis by providers and health plan management. Information used to evaluate accessibility is derived from various reports, such as grievances, referral/utilization, claims/encounters, and sample studies. Aggregation and trending of information is absolutely essential to identify potential problem areas. Providers who fall outside established thresholds or standards of care should be targeted for further study. The results of all quality review activities should be communicated to the clinic or health plan providers. This is necessary for education and for solicitation of suggestions for improvement.

Accessibility-of-care data should be reported to the clinic's or health plan's quality management committee and governing body at least quarterly. This report should include the results of statistical measures of accessibility, a description of all activities designed to improve accessibility, and the effectiveness of improvement activities. A sample format for the statistical portion of this report is shown in figure 11-6.

□ Documenting Quality Improvement

Many different measures can help determine whether a quality review of health care accessibility resulted in improvement. Verified improvements in accessibility may include a documented reduction in patients' waiting time in the physician's office or for an appointment (by type of care needed). If the health care delivery system is an HMO, changes in provider contracts or expectations should mirror the plan's quality thresholds or standards that are established through the review process. Other measures of access improvement are lower out-of-plan costs (noncontracted services) and fewer complaints.

One major area that is frequently scrutinized by the federal and state HMO regulators is the need for adequate geographic coverage by providers. The plans are responsible for providing access to care for their members. Improvements can be documented merely by reporting the geographic coverage of providers. This process is very critical and sometimes is the easiest to document, but may be difficult to attain if providers are unwilling to contract with the health plan.

Figure 11-6. Statistical Portion of a Quarterly Report on Accessibility of Care

Accessibility of Care Quarterly Quality Management Report							
	Data Source					Result of Case Inquiry by Medical Director/QA Committee	
Issue Category	Surveys	Encounter/ Billing	Studies	Complaints and Grievances	Case Reviews	Number Reviewed	Number Considered Inappropriate
Out-of-Plan Referrals							
Medical Record Total Cases Reviewed							
Referral Waiting Times							
Emergent							
Urgent							
Routine							
24-Hour Availability							
Geographic Location							
Caseload							
Patient/Provider Ratios							
Language Requirements							
Total							

☐ Conclusion

Adequate patient access to health care services is the foundation of a quality health care delivery system, whether the system is a private clinic or a health plan. As the number of outpatient health care services increases, the need to implement programs to evaluate and improve quality, including accessibility, will become more important. The evaluation of quality in the ambulatory care setting is a new challenge for many quality management professionals. However, many of the same concepts and techniques used to verify quality of care in a hospital are invaluable in establishing an outpatient quality management program. The major difference is volume. Ambulatory care services are much more abundant than inpatient services, making quality more difficult to monitor, especially when reviewing for accessibility of care. But there are rewards for making the quality commitment. Patients and health plan members are becoming more informed and are paying for a greater share of their health care services. Quality assessment and improvement efforts at the clinic level and within the health plan will be rewarded by satisfied patients who will return to the same ambulatory care facility as they need care.

☐ References

1. Office of Prepaid Health Care. *Health Maintenance Organization (Title XIII) Manual.* Washington, DC: Health Care Financing Administration, Aug. 1989, 24 (4205.4.c).

2. Joint Commission on Accreditation of Healthcare Organizations. *Quality Assurance in Ambulatory Care.* 2nd ed. Chicago: JCAHO, 1990, p. 59.

3. Kaiser, L. R. How to make the mind more receptive to new ideas. *Healthcare Forum* 30(2):51, Mar.–Apr. 1987.

4. Office of Prepaid Health Care. *Quality Assurance Guidelines for Health Maintenance Organizations and Competitive Medical Plans.* Washington, DC: Health Care Financing Administration, July 25, 1986, p. 3 [42 CRF 110.107 (b)(1)].

Section Seven

Evaluation of Patient Satisfaction

As the health care industry embraces the concepts of continuous quality improvement, the need for involving patients in the quality measurement process has become essential. Although the need for quality management in clinical practice is paramount, ambulatory care providers must incorporate patient satisfaction into their quality assessment and improvement activities. Through a knowledge of customer expectations, the ambulatory care organization can design its systems around a "customer-first" orientation. Continuous communication with customers is needed to identify issues of poor quality, customer expectations, and incidents of good quality. This information should shape the organization's quality improvement efforts.

Chapter 12 provides general suggestions on how to design a patient survey questionnaire. The variables that must be considered during survey development and the common pitfalls of measuring patient satisfaction are described. This chapter serves as an introduction to the next two chapters in this section. Chapter 13 presents a patient satisfaction survey process used by one ambulatory care unit. Many of the basic theories of survey design presented in chapter 12 are illustrated in this example. Ideas are also presented for reporting the survey data back to individual ambulatory care departments. In addition to global satisfaction surveys, ambulatory care providers may wish to obtain focused feedback on the quality of care given by a particular problem area. This information is useful as the institution targets opportunities to improve quality and reduce errors, delays, and other such problems. Chapter 14 describes the process used to incorporate patient satisfaction data into the redesign of a large, complex ambulatory care system. By obtaining patient satisfaction data prior to making ambulatory care system changes, the institution became more customer-oriented in its strategic planning and change processes.

Chapter 12

Considerations for the Survey Process

Priscilla Kibbee

I nterest in determining patient satisfaction has greatly intensified in today's competitive health care market. A key component of quality improvement theory is that suppliers of a good or service must receive feedback from consumers in order to identify deficiencies and guide the design of improvement.[1] For this reason, considerable effort has gone into the development of systems to capture patient or customer reactions to their health care experiences.

Hospitals have been forerunners in this endeavor, with the current JCAHO requirements mandating formal mechanisms to handle patient complaints and solicit patient satisfaction information.[2-3] In the ambulatory care setting, measures of patient satisfaction began in earnest with the growth of health maintenance organizations (HMOs) and similar managed care insurance plans. Federally approved HMOs are required to have a quality assurance system in place within their provider organization. An essential component of this quality assurance program is enrollee involvement in satisfaction surveys and a formal grievance procedure.[4] As physicians and other ambulatory care providers joined with federally approved HMOs and similar insurance plans, they became contractually responsible for involvement in these satisfaction survey processes.

In a study reported in 1989, an outpatient setting showed a decline in patients' overall satisfaction. The portion of respondents who said they were "very satisfied" with the quality of their care was 92.3 percent in 1988 and only 85.2 percent in 1989.[5] In examining these responses, the author found the following leading causes of outpatient dissatisfaction:[6]

- A perception of poor quality
- Waiting time while others are treated first
- A perceived lack of care
- Discourteous nurses and staff

Research into patient satisfaction issues has led to the identification of several factors that are thought to affect patients' attitudes about the quality of their health care experience. Variables considered to have a positive or negative influence on the results of patient satisfaction surveys include:

- Age: Older patients tend to report higher levels of satisfaction than do younger patients.[7]
- Gender: Women tend to be more satisfied than men.[8]
- Social class: Satisfaction is greater if the practitioner is of the same socioeconomic class and race.[9]
- Physical and psychological status: The patient's health status prior to receiving any care may cause him or her to be more or less satisfied.[10]
- Patients' attitudes and expectations concerning medical care: A patient who has previously had a bad experience at the health care organization may have negative expectations.[11]
- In psychiatric settings: This variable has to do with the client's degree of optimism about treatment of mental illness and his or her chances for readjustment.[12]
- The health care organization's structure and financing of care: Patients with higher out-of-pocket costs tend to be less satisfied than those whose insurance plan covers more expenses.[13]
- Cost of care: The higher the cost, the lower the level of patient satisfaction.[14]
- Accessibility, availability, and convenience of care: The lower the frustration level in gaining access to care, the higher the level of satisfaction.[15]
- Perceived competence of providers: Satisfaction is related to patients' perceptions of technical skills, intelligence, and qualifications, although perceived interpersonal and communication skills generally account for more of the variation in patient satisfaction.[16]
- Perceived improvement in health: Although this is a predictor of patient satisfaction, it has not been extensively addressed.[17-18]
- Perceived kindness of providers: Good communication skills, empathy, and caring: These are all high-ranking on lists of patients' expectations and on their subsequent level of satisfaction.[19]

Researchers have also suggested factors that limit the validity of patient satisfaction survey results:[20]

- Patients lack the knowledge to accurately assess the technical competence of medical personnel. Furthermore, their physical or emotional status can easily impede judgment.
- Patients are influenced by "nonmedical" factors such as the provider's interpersonal skills. A good bedside manner can easily mask doubtful technical quality.
- Patients are often reluctant to disclose what they really think because of their sense of dependency or prior failures in patient–physician communication.
- Patients cannot accurately recall aspects of the delivery process. Moreover, patient surveys, or even face-to-face interviews, are imperfect means for measuring highly subjective phenomena.

Although researchers have identified many different variables that affect patients' satisfaction with health care services and the limitations that influence the validity of survey techniques, ambulatory care providers must overcome these obstacles and forge ahead in their quest to measure patient satisfaction. The principles of quality improvement, which include a customer-first orientation, require that customer satisfaction be constantly sought out and incorporated into the improvement phases of quality management. Ambulatory care facilities must be aware of previous research findings and use this information to design and implement a patient satisfaction feedback process that meets their quality measurement requirements and allows for useful expression of their customers' service contentment. Following are some general guidelines for developing a patient satisfaction survey.

☐ The Survey Tool

In the process of developing the survey instrument, the following determinations need to be made: delineation of service encounter areas, identification of topologies of satisfaction or dimensions of care for each service encounter, and determination of the survey's measurement rankings. Each of these components is discussed in the following sections.

Service Encounter Areas

To design a facility-specific survey, start by looking at the ambulatory care process and breaking down each step in the service cycle. Each step has a discrete beginning and end. The survey should be designed to allow customers to rate each discrete service encounter. Steiber and Krowinski suggest that viewing the patient's experience as a series of service encounters helps the provider "recognize where any given department's responsibilities are most readily identified, evaluated, and remolded."[21]

A list of service encounter areas for an ambulatory care clinic would include:

- Clinic location and appointments
- Clinic building, offices, and waiting time
- Clinic assistants and helpers
- Physicians
- Health services offered
- Service results

By requesting patient feedback regarding the quality of each distinct ambulatory care service area (rather than general questions covering all services), the provider has better information on which to make improvement changes in areas found to be problems. Be certain to design the patient satisfaction survey in such a way that each service encounter area is evaluated individually.

Dimensions of Care

There are numerous categories, or dimensions, of patient satisfaction that evaluate a finite dimension of care. Those most frequently measured are the personal aspects of care, the technical quality of care, accessibility and availability of care, continuity of care, patient convenience, physical setting, financial considerations, and efficacy. The ambulatory care provider must determine for each service encounter area which of these categories/dimensions to evaluate. This is an individual provider choice, based on the objectives of the survey and physical limitations of the survey tool. By adding the measurement dimensions to each clinic service encounter area, the patient questionnaire begins to take shape. Following are some examples:[22]

- Clinic location and appointments:
  —Location
  —Parking
  —Hours of operation
  —Obtained appointments
  —Obtained desired appointment time(s)
- Clinic building, offices, and waiting time:
  —Amount of waiting time
  —Appearance of building, office, and waiting areas
  —Comfort of offices and waiting areas
  —Appearance and clarity of signs, posted instructions, and announcements

155

- Clinic assistants and helpers:
  —Courtesy and helpfulness of telephone operators, receptionists, and medical assistants
- Physicians:
  —Skill
  —Friendliness
  —Clarity of information and advice
  —Thoroughness
  —Amount of time spent
- Health services offered:
  —Received the desired services
  —Saw the desired nurse or physician
- Service results:
  —Success of services
  —Speed of services
  —Value of services
  —Usefulness of information and advice

Rankings

Several options are available for classifying satisfaction scores. Feedback is better if the customer is given more than two answer choices, that is, more than "yes" or "no."[23] Ware and Hays, in studies of patient satisfaction with outpatient visits, found "excellent–poor" ratings superior to direct satisfaction ratings like "very satisfied–not at all satisfied."[24]

Quality ratings, such as the following, provide useful information:

( ) Poor
( ) Fair
( ) Average
( ) Good
( ) Excellent

Occurrence ratings measure the frequency of a desired event or the consistency of a desired action. A scale with either three or five choices can be used:

( ) Infrequently   ( ) Never
( ) Sometimes   ( ) Seldom
( ) Always   ( ) Sometimes
                    ( ) Almost always
                    ( ) Always

Agreement scales are used to measure the respondent's consensus with a statement. An example of an agreement rating is provided below:

( ) Strongly disagree
( ) Disagree
( ) Neutral
( ) Agree
( ) Strongly agree

Expectation ratings can apply to both quality and the occurrence of certain standards. To measure a patient's expectations, use the following phrases:[25]

( ) Much worse than I expected
( ) Worse than I expected
( ) As I expected
( ) Better than I expected
( ) Much better than I expected

Notice that all of these scales are composed of an odd number of components—three or five. With an even number, such as two or four, there is no neutral point, and the respondent is forced into a negative or positive stance, skewing the results—for example, never, seldom, almost always, always. In cases where even-numbered scales have a neutral position, then either the negative or positive side is given more weight—for example, never, seldom, sometimes, always. Here there are two possible negative answers, one neutral and one positive. A sample patient questionnaire, constructed to evaluate the dimensions of clinic services previously described, is shown in figure 12-1.

Additional Information

When one recalls the variables that affect patient satisfaction with health care services, discussed earlier in the chapter, it is important to include space on the survey tool for patients to add demographic and other pertinent data: for example, age, sex, race, type of insurance plan, and so forth. These data elements can later be used by the ambulatory care provider in the analysis of survey results. Stratifying the results by these important variables may show patterns that would not be evident in the general survey population.

☐ Survey Methodology

Careful planning is necessary to ensure that the patient satisfaction survey yields meaningful information for the outpatient clinic. Sampling, data collection methods, and survey format should be thought out very carefully in the early stages of the process. Following are several preliminary questions related to data collection and survey format that can help guide the development and planning stages:[26]

Sampling and data collection method

1. Will all the patients served by the facility at a given time be represented by the survey sample population?
2. Is the sample size adequate?
3. Will the data collection method ensure the response rate desired?

These questions are addressed during the survey design process described in the following two chapters. In general, the ambulatory care provider should attempt to gather patient feedback from no less than 5 percent of its annual population.[27]

Survey format

1. Do the questions address the aspects of care and service that patients perceive as most important?
2. Will the questions and rating scale yield reliable and valid results?

Again, these issues are addressed by Disch and Moir in subsequent chapters. One method for ensuring a "yes" answer to each of these questions is to pilot-test the survey tool with a small sample of patients. It is better to identify problem areas early in the survey process before a large number of inadequately designed questionnaires are released to all patients.

☐ Conclusion

The customer-oriented ambulatory care provider must keep constantly informed of its patients' perceptions of quality. This requires a concerted effort to obtain feedback that

Figure 12-1. Outpatient Satisfaction Survey Form

May we have your comments, please?

Your opinions about the _____ (name of facility or service) are our guide to better service, so please take a few minutes to fill out this questionnaire.

When completed, please place it in the questionnaire box at the desk.

Clinic location and appointments

	Excellent	Good	Fair	Poor
Location	☐	☐	☐	☐
Parking facilities	☐	☐	☐	☐
Hours of operation	☐	☐	☐	☐
Ease of obtaining appointments	☐	☐	☐	☐

Clinic building and offices

	Excellent	Good	Fair	Poor
Appearance of building, offices, and waiting areas	☐	☐	☐	☐
Comfort of offices and waiting areas	☐	☐	☐	☐
Appearance and clarity of signs, posted instructions, and announcements	☐	☐	☐	☐

Waiting time

The amount of time you had to wait for your appointment today was _____ minutes. The amount of time you usually wait is _____.

Is the amount of waiting time acceptable? _____

Unacceptable? _____ What items could have been provided to make your wait more pleasurable? _____

_____

Clinic staff

Courtesy and helpfulness of telephone operators and receptionists	☐	☐	☐	☐

Primary therapist

Please rate the *primary* person you saw on this visit (physician, nurse, social worker, and so on).

The primary person seen was a _____.

Skill	☐	☐	☐	☐
Friendliness	☐	☐	☐	☐
Clarity of information and advice	☐	☐	☐	☐
Thoroughness	☐	☐	☐	☐

The amount of time spent with you was enough to satisfy your needs today.

_____ Yes   _____ No

If no, what did you need that was not received? _____

_____

Did you see the staff member you wished to see?

_____ Yes   _____ No

If not, what was the explanation for the change? _____

_____

Service results

Do you feel that the services we provide are a good value for the cost?

_____ Yes   _____ No

If not, please comment on the reason: _____

_____

Have you found the information and advice we gave you to be useful?

_____ Yes   _____ No

If not, please comment on the reason: _____

_____

Figure 12-1. (Continued)

Are there any additional comments you would like to make?

_____

_____

_____

_____

If you like, we would be happy to discuss some of your answers further with you. If so, please include your name, address, and telephone number. Thank you again for taking the time to help us maintain a high level of quality care.

Name: _____ Address: _____

Telephone number: _____ Best time to call _____

is useful in making necessary improvements in ambulatory care services. Except for those who are familiar with the technical aspects of outpatient health care services, most patients do not know what constitutes clinical professional competence. Therefore, patient surveys must focus on the quality of the interaction between the care provider and the recipient—sometimes termed the "quality of behavior."[28]

By identifying what patients want from a facility, both in the quality of behavior and the quality of technical expertise, the effective preparation strategy is to design health care systems that place the customer first. To solicit meaningful feedback from patients, ambulatory care providers must concern themselves with several factors inherent in any survey process: survey design and question validity, sample size, distribution, and relevance of answers.

☐ References

1. Rubin, H. R. Patient evaluations of hospital care: a review of the literature. _Medical Care_ 28(9):S3, Sept. 1990.

2. Joint Commission on Accreditation of Healthcare Organizations. Standards on management of patient complaints—AMH, AHCSM, LTCSM. _Joint Commission Perspectives_ 9(5/6):12–14, May–June 1989.

3. Joint Commission on Accreditation of Healthcare Organizations. Revised CSM standards address patient complaints. _Joint Commission Perspectives_ 10(1):8–9, Jan.–Feb. 1990.

4. Office of Prepaid Health Care. _Quality Assurance Guidelines for Health Maintenance Organizations and Competitive Medical Plans._ Washington, DC: Department of Health and Human Services, 1986.

5. Eubanks, P. Patient satisfaction levels decline slightly in 1989. _Hospitals_ 64(16):43, Aug. 20, 1989.

6. Eubanks, P. Outpatient care: a nationwide revolution. _Hospitals_ 64(15):28–35, Aug. 5, 1990.

7. Cleary, P., and McNeil, B. Patient satisfaction as an indicator of quality care. _Inquiry_ 25(1):25–36, Spring 1988.

8. Cleary and McNeil, pp. 25–36.

9. Cleary and McNeil, pp. 25–36.

10. Pascoe, G., and Attkisson, C. The evaluation ranking scale: a new methodology for assessing satisfaction. _Evaluation and Program Planning_ 6:335–46, 1983.

11. McMillan, J. Measuring consumer satisfaction to improve quality of care. _Health Progress_ 68(2):54–55, 76–80, Mar. 1987.

12. Distefano, M. K., Jr., Pryer, M. W., and Garrison, J. L. Attitudinal, demographic, and outcome correlates of clients' satisfaction. *Psychological Reports* 47(1):287–89, Aug. 1980.

13. Elliot, T., Dunaye, T., and Jounson, P. Determining patient satisfaction in a Medicare health maintenance organization. *Journal of Ambulatory Care Management* 14(1):34–46, Jan. 1991.

14. Elliot and others, pp. 34–46.

15. Pascoe, G. Patient satisfaction in primary health care: a literature review and analysis. *Evaluation and Program Planning* 6:185–210, 1983.

16. Woolley, F. R., and others. The effects of doctor-patient communication on satisfaction and outcome of care. *Social Science and Medicine* 12:123–28, 1978.

17. Fleming, G. V. Hospital structure and consumer satisfaction. *Health Services Research* 16:43–63, 1981.

18. Benson, D., and Miller, J. *Quality Assurance for Primary Care Centers.* Indianapolis: Methodist Hospitals of Indiana, Inc., 1988, p. 20.

19. Cleary and McNeil, pp. 25–36.

20. Vuori, H. Patient satisfaction—an attribute or indicator of the quality of care? *Quality Review Bulletin* 13(3):106–8, Mar. 1987.

21. Steiber, S. How consumers rate health care quality. *Health Care Strategic Management* 6(8):6–8, Aug. 1988.

22. Elliot and others, pp. 34–46.

23. Oliver, R. Measurement and evaluation of satisfaction process in retail services. *Journal of Retailing* 57(4):25–48, Apr. 1981.

24. Ware, J. E., and Hays, R. D. Methods for measuring patient satisfaction with specific medical encounters. *Medical Care* 9:43, Sept. 1986.

25. Peterson, K. *The Strategic Approach to Quality Service in Health Care.* Rockville, MD: Aspen Publishers, 1988, p. 166.

26. Nelson, E., Hays, R., Larson, C., and Batalden, P. The patient judgment system: reliability and validity. *Quality Review Bulletin* 15(6):185–91, June 1989.

27. Joint Commission on Accreditation of Healthcare Organizations. *Quality Assurance in Managed Care.* Chicago: JCAHO, 1989, p. 161.

28. King, C. A. Service quality is different. *Quality Progress* 18(6):14, 1985.

Chapter 13

A Global Patient Satisfaction Tool for Ambulatory Care Services

Cathy Disch

Developing a useful patient satisfaction survey is always a challenging task, but it can be even more challenging in a complex ambulatory care environment. This chapter details the development and implementation of the survey process in a large health care system and provides examples of the project timetable, the survey that was used, and the format for displaying survey results.

The University of Texas Medical Branch (UTMB) in Galveston is one of 15 components of the University of Texas System. The UTMB occupies 64 acres on the eastern end of Galveston Island and includes 71 major buildings housing four medical schools, two institutes, a sophisticated health care complex, numerous research facilities, and varied support services. These include seven hospitals, a major medical library, classroom buildings, specialty centers, extensive research laboratories, maintenance areas, and office buildings.

John Sealy Hospital, with its 12-story, 528-bed tower and 22-room surgical suite, is the hub of the UTMB Hospitals' patient care complex of seven hospitals and 85 outpatient clinics. Adult outpatient services are centralized in the seven-story Ambulatory Care Center (ACC), while those for children are in the Child Health Center. Services for more than 250,000 patient visits are provided annually in the clinics.

☐ Quality Review Background

On April 1, 1990, UT-MED, The Group Practice of Medicine at UTMB, assumed management responsibility for the outpatient clinics. Under the direction of a new administrator, the ACC and the outpatient areas became an integral partner in support of the mission and evolving goals of UT-MED to upgrade the quality of outpatient services and institute more efficient clinic operations.

To accomplish these goals, a patient satisfaction survey was proposed as a means of assessing current operations and perceptions of clinic services. With the approval of the annual budget in June 1990, this objective was formalized in the Ambulatory Service Department plan for the coming year. Initiation of the patient satisfaction survey project was planned for September 1, 1990.

In addition to the goal of improving the quality and efficiency of clinic services, other project objectives were:

- To establish baseline data to measure the effects of changes in service on patient and staff perceptions
- To identify positive results for recognizing people and achievements
- To identify areas where improvements are needed or opportunities exist to strengthen overall service provided
- To integrate patient satisfaction into an overall quality improvement program that includes referring physicians, employees, and all clinic staff

The patient satisfaction survey project, then, is just one component of a service excellence strategy to guide clinic operations, decision making, and planning.

☐ The Patient Satisfaction Survey Project

Prior to the actual start of the project on September 1, a number of decisions had to be made to define the focus and timing of the project.

Initial Planning Stage

The administrator assigned clinic administrative directors as the project team and charged it with defining the scope of the survey, identifying resources needed, and determining the time frame for completion. A decision was made to develop an internal survey format and reporting mechanism rather than purchase an existing survey package. The team felt strongly that a purchased product would not provide the information specific to UTMB services, the flexibility to produce ad hoc reports, or the ability to change future survey content if desired.

During the month of August the project team completed its assignment. One of its tasks was to define the scope of the survey, and the team knew that patients at UTMB represented diverse cultures, educational levels, and economic backgrounds. As in other academic medical centers, some patients are seen in a private-practice setting by faculty, but the majority of patients are seen by resident physicians in staff clinics supervised by faculty. After thorough discussion of patient and institutional factors, the scope of the survey was determined to include all clinic patients. The primary goal, on which the project schedule was based, was to complete the patient portion of the survey process during the fourth quarter of 1990. Therefore, this meant the questionnaire development and printing had to be done quickly. Data entry, final reporting, and project evaluation could then occur during the first quarter of 1991. Although the clinic staff would be responsible for the distribution and administration of the survey, additional resources would be needed for programming, reporting, and data entry. Major tasks to complete the project were identified and a formal plan to implement the survey, including a timetable, was determined. Figure 13-1 summarizes the plan and the timetable.

Survey Development

With the initial planning completed and the scope of the survey determined, the development of the survey was the next step. The existing patient complaint process provided an initial guide to identifying criteria to include in the survey questionnaire. Interviews with the medical staff, managers, and clinic employees provided further input. The patient and institutional factors discussed in the preliminary planning stages were taken into consideration during the criteria development stage.

Figure 13-1. Formal Survey Plan and Timetable

Action Steps	Duration	Dates
Perform Preliminary Planning	30 days	(8/1–8/31)
—Assign project team		
—Define project scope		
—Identify resources		
—Determine plan/time frame		
Begin Project	30 weeks	(9/1–4/1/90)
—Questionnaire development	6 weeks	(9/4–10/12)
—Survey logistics	6 weeks	(9/10–10/26)
—Determination of Survey dates	1 week	(10/15)
—Programming development	12 weeks	(9/17–12/7)
—Data entry	6 weeks	(12/2–1/11)
—Report production	2 weeks	(1/21–2/1)
—Data analysis	3 weeks	(2/4–2/22)
—Final report distribution	2 weeks	(3/4–3/15)
—Feedback and evaluation	2 weeks	(3/18–3/29)

The results of the interviews and data gathering from the complaint process focused on five major areas of assessment:

1. Access to services
2. Courtesy/concern for patients
3. Amenities
4. Overall care
5. Delays in service

These five areas were then developed into survey questions that were listed appropriately under each patient contact point during a clinic visit. As a result, the flow of the questionnaire mirrored the patients' progress through their clinic visit, beginning with making an appointment and finishing with billing questions. The completed questionnaire, as shown in figure 13-2, included the following patient contact points:

- Appointment-making process
- Parking and signage
- Check-in process
- Waiting area
- Nursing staff
- Medical staff
- Diagnostic services
- Billing services

To further assess patient needs and assist management in analyzing the data and recommending change, six additional questions were included (these are questions 9–14 in sections III and IV of figure 13-2). Finally, patients were asked, "What *one* thing could have made your experience at the UTMB outpatient clinics a better one?"

Figure 13-2. Patient Satisfaction Survey Instrument

Welcome to the University of Texas Medical Branch (UTMB) outpatient clinics. All the members of our staff are dedicated to providing excellent health care and responsive service. Your honest opinions about your experiences here help us determine how well we are meeting this goal and provide us with the information necessary to make improvements or changes. Please take a few minutes to complete and return this survey.

Directions: Please answer the following questions by checking the answer that best describes your most recent outpatient clinic visit to UTMB.

I. BEFORE YOUR APPOINTMENT

1. Appointment-Making Process

   a. When you called for an appointment, which type of appointment did you request?
   ( ) Urgent
   ( ) Routine

   b. If you requested an urgent appointment, how soon after you called for an appointment did the actual appointment take place?
   ( ) Within 24 hours
   ( ) Within 48 hours
   ( ) Over 48 hours
   ( ) Does not apply

   c. If you requested a routine appointment, how soon after you called for an appointment did the actual appointment take place?
   ( ) Within 2 weeks
   ( ) 2–4 weeks
   ( ) 1–2 months
   ( ) Over 2 months
   ( ) Does not apply

   d. How would you grade this time period?
   ( ) Excellent
   ( ) Good
   ( ) Average
   ( ) Poor

   e. Were you treated courteously by the person making your appointment?
   ( ) Yes
   ( ) No

   f. Did you request to see a specific physician?
   ( ) Yes
   ( ) No

   g. Did you receive an appointment with the physician of your choice?
   ( ) Yes
   ( ) No

   h. How would you grade the appointment-making process?
   ( ) Excellent
   ( ) Good
   ( ) Average
   ( ) Poor

II. THE DAY OF YOUR APPOINTMENT

2. Parking and Signage

   a. Were you able to find a parking space easily?
   ( ) Yes
   ( ) No
   ( ) Does not apply

   b. If you needed a wheelchair, was one available?
   ( ) Yes
   ( ) No
   ( ) Does not apply

   c. Were the directions to the parking garage clear?
   ( ) Yes
   ( ) No
   ( ) Does not apply

   d. Was the building where your clinic appointment was located easy to find?
   ( ) Yes
   ( ) No
   ( ) Does not apply

   e. Was the clinic easy to locate once you were in the building?
   ( ) Yes
   ( ) No
   ( ) Does not apply

   f. How would you grade the parking facilities?
   ( ) Excellent
   ( ) Good
   ( ) Average
   ( ) Poor

Figure 13-2. (Continued)

g. How would you grade the directional signs around UTMB?
( ) Excellent
( ) Good
( ) Average
( ) Poor

3. Check-in Process

a. Were you treated courteously by the staff in the reception area?
( ) Yes
( ) No

b. Did you encounter any delays in the check-in process?
( ) Yes
( ) No

c. Was the check-in process easy to understand?
( ) Yes
( ) No

d. How would you grade the check-in process?
( ) Excellent
( ) Good
( ) Average
( ) Poor

4. Waiting Area

a. Was there enough seating in the waiting room?
( ) Yes
( ) No

b. Was the waiting room attractive in its decor?
( ) Yes
( ) No

c. Was the seating comfortable?
( ) Yes
( ) No

d. Was the waiting room clean?
( ) Yes
( ) No

e. Was there someone available to answer your questions or provide information?
( ) Yes
( ) No
( ) Does not apply

f. How would you rate the waiting room facility?
( ) Excellent
( ) Good
( ) Average
( ) Poor

5. Nursing Staff

a. Were you treated courteously by the nursing staff?
( ) Yes
( ) No

b. Were your questions to the nurse answered to your satisfaction?
( ) Yes
( ) No
( ) Does not apply

c. Were the instructions you received from the nurse clear?
( ) Yes
( ) No
( ) Does not apply

d. How would you rate the nursing staff?
( ) Excellent
( ) Good
( ) Average
( ) Poor

6. Medical Staff

a. Did the physician treat you courteously?
( ) Yes
( ) No

b. Did your physician examine you in a reasonable amount of time?
( ) Yes
( ) No

c. Were the questions you asked your physician answered to your satisfaction?
( ) Yes
( ) No
( ) Does not apply

(continued on next page)

Figure 13-2. (Continued)

d. Were your condition and treatment explained clearly to you?

( ) Yes
( ) No

e. How would you grade your physician?

( ) Excellent
( ) Good
( ) Average
( ) Poor

7. Diagnostic Services (X rays, laboratory services, and so forth)

a. Did you receive adequate instructions on where to go for your test(s)?

( ) Yes
( ) No
( ) Does not apply

b. Was the procedure(s) performed at the scheduled time?

( ) Yes
( ) No
( ) Does not apply

c. Were you treated courteously by the staff?

( ) Yes
( ) No
( ) Does not apply

d. Was the procedure(s) explained fully to you?

( ) Yes
( ) No
( ) Does not apply

e. How would you grade the diagnostic services?

( ) Excellent
( ) Good
( ) Average
( ) Poor

If you underwent diagnostic testing, please indicate the test(s) you had performed:

8. Physicians' Billing Service (Your responses to the following questions should be based on your past experiences.)

a. Was your bill easy to understand?

( ) Yes
( ) No
( ) Does not apply

b. Were the charges correct?

( ) Yes
( ) No
( ) Does not apply

c. Were your questions to the Physicians' Billing Service staff answered to your satisfaction?

( ) Yes
( ) No
( ) Does not apply

d. Were you treated courteously by the Physicians' Billing Service staff?

( ) Yes
( ) No
( ) Does not apply

d. How would you grade the Physicians' Billing Service?

( ) Excellent
( ) Good
( ) Average
( ) Poor

III. OVERALL SATISFACTION

9. Overall, how would you grade the care and treatment you received in the UTMB outpatient clinics?

( ) Excellent
( ) Good
( ) Average
( ) Poor

10. Would you return to UTMB for your future medical treatment?

( ) Yes
( ) No

11. Would you recommend UTMB to others?

( ) Yes
( ) No

IV. OTHER INFORMATION

12. Was this your first visit to the UTMB outpatient clinics?

( ) Yes
( ) No

Figure 13-2. (Continued)

13. Please check the reasons why you chose UTMB clinics for your medical care.

( ) Physician ability
( ) Location
( ) Reputation for quality care
( ) Referred by another physician
( ) Past experience at UTMB
Other (please identify):

14. Are you an UTMB employee?

( ) Yes
( ) No

V. RECOMMENDATIONS

15. What *one* thing could have made your experience at the UTMB outpatient clinics a better one?

Response Scoring

The scoring system was intended to be a simple grading system for the patient. Answers were either *yes/no* or on a scale of *excellent, good, average, poor*. Write-in items were limited to two, one of which was the recommendation question just mentioned (that is, What could have made your experience better?). The project team was primarily interested in obtaining a consistent format in order to compare all the patient contact points, provide a constant data entry format, and be easy for the patient to understand and complete.

Survey Layout

The layout, as previously discussed, was developed to follow the patient flow process. Designers were consulted to assist with the reading level and blocking of the question-and-answer areas. Shading of main headings, type style, color, and paper selection were discussed and decided on. A three-page foldout design was selected as the format because it would include all the questions, provide a pleasing uncluttered document, allow the form to be used as a self-mailer, and serve as the data entry document.

Sample Size

Once the survey process was established, the goal of the Ambulatory Services Department was to complete two patient survey cycles during one year, with the survey cycle period lasting two weeks. This method was chosen because it would maximize survey exposure to a greater number of clinic patients than a phone or mail survey and provide management with more valid feedback. However, this would not preclude a focused survey on a particular patient population, if desired.

Average daily and weekly visit counts were easily determined for the individual clinic areas. The return rate goal for the initial survey period was set at 15 percent of patient visits. The distribution of questionnaires to the patients was expected to vary depending on the check-in flow. It was anticipated that only one-third of all patients would receive a questionnaire to complete because the clinic admitting area is very busy and staff would not have time to explain the survey to each patient.

Method of Distribution

A supply of questionnaires was prestamped with the individual clinic name and provided to the clinic director for distribution by the clinic staff. Additional surveys were available if needed. During the actual survey period, a pencil and the survey were given to the patient at check-in with verbal instructions on how to complete the survey. Clinic staff encouraged patients to complete the survey and were available to assist them if questions arose. Survey return boxes were strategically located throughout the clinics as well as in the pharmacy and at exit doors from the building. A small number of patients took the survey home, completed it, and mailed it back.

Clinic staff also maintained logs during the two-week period to track the surveys. Specific data gathered included number of patient visits, number of surveys distributed, and number of completed surveys. Return rates were calculated using these data.

☐ Survey Data Compilation

Data entry of the survey results was assigned to a primary data entry clerk with backup provided by an additional employee. The surveys were automatically numbered by the computer program as a tracking and counting mechanism. The clerks batched and entered the data by clinic. The clerks also maintained a log to track their project hours. The programmer provided initial training to the clerks once the program was loaded on a personal computer in the department.

Computer assistance and programming were provided by a programmer from the Academic Computing Department. The programmer chosen had previous patient survey experience and was familiar with the clinic environment. The tasks to be completed in this phase included writing the program, testing the program and reporting, training the data entry staff, printing the reports, and reviewing and correcting program errors. The software program was developed using D-Base™ with assistance from CLIPPER™ in compiling the response data. The programmer worked closely with a project leader in developing the program once the questionnaire content and layout were approved.

Two critical concerns in this phase of project development were ease of data entry and reporting. Input screens were designed to replicate the survey. Quality checks were included to prevent input errors and ensure correct data for reporting.

The reports were developed in consultation with administration. Reporting was required for each clinic area in addition to an overall summary of data for all clinics. Staff patient visits and faculty patient visits were to be reported separately.

☐ Survey Results

A complete analysis of the patient survey project includes not only the information obtained from the patients, but also an evaluation of the survey process itself.

The Survey Process

The early phases of the survey process went well, up to and including completion of the survey tool. The overwhelming number of surveys completed—twice the anticipated number—caused a delay in the data entry process and outcome reporting. A total of 5,041 surveys were distributed to clinic patients. This was 54 percent of the total number of patients seen during the survey period. Of those who received the survey, 2,903 patients completed and returned them for a return rate of 58 percent. The goal to survey 15 percent of patients seen was exceeded. The actual percentage was 31 percent.

Data entry was completed three weeks later than scheduled, even with additional clerical staff. Report production was not completed until late March 1991. The final format of the reports was modified to provide a better display of the data and thus improve analysis, as well as to provide a more professional presentation to readers. (See figure 13-3 for format sample.) As a result, final report distribution occurred one month later than planned.

Upon completion of the reports, the information was distributed to the clinic medical directors and staff of the 15 clinics surveyed. In addition, ancillary and support service areas (for example, pharmacy and billing) were provided with the results for their departments. Reports were presented to the medical staff executive committee, board of directors, and the ambulatory care subcommittee. The ambulatory care subcommittee, responsible for overall management of the clinics, set a 90 percent satisfaction level as the quality standard.

Final feedback and evaluation have not occurred. There are, however, a number of improvements that have already been planned for the next survey cycle:

- The surveys will be printed in Spanish for distribution to the clinic's large Hispanic population. It was originally anticipated that clinic staff would be able

Figure 13-3. Sample Page of Report Showing Final Format

		All Staff and Faculty Clinics		All Faculty Clinics		All Staff Clinics	
		#	%	#	%	#	%
1. Accessibility							
a. Were you able to find a parking space easily:	Yes	1,540	55	282	55	1,258	54
	No	944	33	143	28	801	35
	N/A	335	12	84	17	251	11
b. If you needed a wheelchair, was one available?	Yes	495	19	45	10	450	20
	No	191	7	20	5	171	8
	N/A	1,963	74	381	85	1,582	72
c. Were the directions to the parking garage clear?	Yes	1,745	63	270	55	1,475	65
	No	305	11	54	11	251	11
	N/A	730	26	169	34	561	24
d. Was the building where your clinic appointment was located easy to find?	Yes	2,597	91.5	418	83	2,179	93
	No	151	5.5	35	7	116	5
	N/A	94	3	52	10	42	2
e. Was the clinic easy to locate once you were in the building?	Yes	2,619	93	438	86	2,181	95
	No	115	4	24	5	91	4
	N/A	78	3	47	9	31	1
f. How would you grade our parking facilities?	Excellent	534	20	92	20	442	20
	Good	961	36	158	33	803	36.5
	Average	737	27	110	23	627	28.5
	Poor	446	17	113	24	333	15
g. How would you grade the directional signs around UTMB?	Excellent	787	28	82	16.5	705	31
	Good	1,275	46	230	47	1,045	45
	Average	546	19.5	110	22	436	19
	Poor	184	6.5	72	14.5	112	5
2. Check-in Process							
a. Were you treated courteously by the staff in the reception area?	Yes	2,770	97	507	99	2,263	97
	No	83	3	7	1	76	3
b. Did you encounter any delays in the check-in process?	Yes	571	20	77	15	494	22
	No	2,222	80	436	85	1,786	78

to assist patients with translations, if needed, but due to the large number of respondents and the impact on patient flow, this did not occur.

- Improvements will address the fact that not all patients answered all questions. After reviewing the responses, it was determined that the questions most frequently left unanswered were under the foldout page of the questionnaire. Either a different report format or better instructions to the patients will solve this problem.

Patient Information

Overall satisfaction with clinic services was rated as excellent or good (88 percent), with courtesy and concern for patients given high marks (97 percent). The three remaining major assessment areas—delays in service (billing and pharmacy), access to services (parking and signage), and amenities (waiting rooms)—were identified as opportunities for improvement (see figure 13-4) because they failed to achieve at least a 90 percent overall satisfaction rating.

Other findings revealed that 97 percent of all respondents would return to UTMB and would recommend UTMB to others. Patients' reasons for choosing UTMB clinics were also analyzed, and the results are displayed in figure 13-5.

☐ Future Goals

The next three steps to be taken in analyzing the feedback from this patient survey process include the following:

1. Set performance standards for patient satisfaction levels using this survey as baseline data. This will provide a measure against which to compare the impact of changes made.

Figure 13-4. Graph Showing Overall Patient Satisfaction Levels

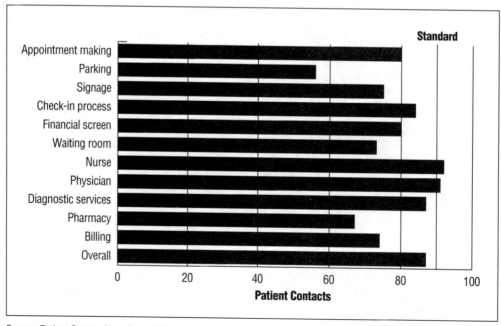

Source: Patient Survey, Nov.–Dec. 1990.

Figure 13-5. Pie Chart Showing Patients' Reasons for Choosing UTMB Clinics

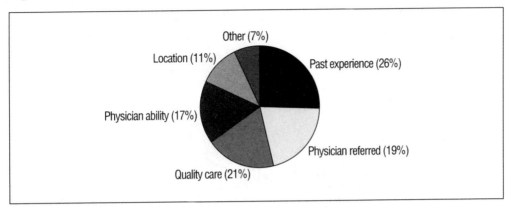

Source: Patient Survey, Nov.–Dec. 1990.

2. Review and explore the survey data by the individual clinic areas so as to identify clinic-specific successes, areas for improvement, and action plans to be incorporated into the quality improvement goals.
3. Plan for the next survey cycle and set a target date for its completion.

After finalizing these steps, a departmentwide response to the survey in the form of a formalized action plan can be developed and integrated with the overall service excellence strategy so as to improve the quality of outpatient services and institute more efficient and satisfying clinic operations.

☐ Conclusion

Both participants and clinic management feel strongly that the patient survey process achieved its original objectives. There were some adjustments made along the way and work is yet to be done, but a successful process has been developed that can be established as an integral part of ongoing ambulatory care operations and an indicator of success.

Chapter 14

A Focused Satisfaction Study of Patient Waiting Times

Beverley J. Moir

R esults from patient satisfaction surveys can be used to redesign delivery systems so that they provide better patient care and customer service and meet customer needs. This chapter describes how dissatisfaction with patient waiting times led to a more efficient approach at The Hospital for Sick Children in Toronto, Canada.

In the large and complex teaching hospital setting of The Hospital for Sick Children, the Ambulatory Services management team did not have accurate or objective data about the amount of time patients and families spend when they come to the hospital for clinic visits. The difficulty in acquiring this information was compounded by the large volume of patients seen on a daily basis. Each day, between 600 and 1,000 patients register for ambulatory care services, and the clinics operate in geographically disparate locations of the hospital under decentralized administrations.

☐ Problem Statement and Project Purpose

The need to develop a system to objectively monitor patients' clinic service became evident in the fall of 1989. Patients and their families were registering complaints about long waits, interaction with overworked and harassed clinic staff, and seemingly short times with physicians after what seemed like inordinately long waiting times. The hospital president regularly received letters or phone calls of complaint from irate families. The general picture of clinic operations was one of disorganization. Waiting rooms were overcrowded, examination rooms were full, staff and physicians looked frustrated, and there were few smiling, friendly faces. There were many opinions circulating throughout the hospital as to how long patients and families had to wait for clinic services. There were equally as many subjective conclusions drawn as to the reasons for these supposedly excessive waits.

The author would like to acknowledge the assistance of Dr. Robert Ehrlich, medical coordinator, Ambulatory Services, and clinical division head of endocrinology, Department of Pediatrics, The Hospital for Sick Children, at the time this chapter was written, and Mrs. Patti Walter, R.N., who was seconded to be the coordinator of the service time study.

As a result, the medical coordinator of ambulatory care services and the director of ambulatory care services hired external consultants to assist in developing and pilot-testing a repeatable system to objectively monitor patients' waiting times. This was done in order to determine where delays were occurring. In approaching the task, it was recognized that simplicity and ease of implementation were extremely important for the following reasons:

- Many people were involved in a patient's visit to the hospital, and therefore large numbers of people would have to be involved in the monitoring system.
- The pattern of visits among physicians and patients was highly variable, and disruption to clinic operations would have to be kept to a minimum.
- It was desirable that broad indicators be developed that would be measurable on a repeated basis and could provide meaningful comparisons across major clinic groupings.

☐ Development of the Service Time Measurement System

The consultants developed and pilot-tested the service time tracking system. It was then used by a senior clinic nurse, who was selected to coordinate the service time tracking project for the three-month period from January to April, 1990. During an eight-week period in early 1990, the service times for the patients attending general pediatric, pediatric specialty, and surgical specialty clinics were surveyed. The decision was made to limit the measurement of the service times to these three broad clinical areas because they alone accounted for approximately 90,000 patient visits per year.

A service time tracking form (see figure 14-1) was developed for recording individual patients' demographic information as well as their movement and times throughout the ambulatory care clinic visit. The form was designed to capture patients' arrival and departure times, and how and where their time was spent in between these two times. Custom-designed software using FoxBase™ was developed for the project for use on Macintosh™ hardware. The program was developed to produce summary reports for individual clinics, roll-up (summary) reports for clinical divisions, and a general summary report showing clinic service time activity in the general pediatric, medical specialty, and surgical specialty areas. Details about the content of the reports are provided later in this chapter. Definitions were required to ensure consistency of terminology and of measurement approach; they are listed in figure 14-2 (p. 176).

☐ System Implementation

The project coordinator (the senior clinical nurse previously mentioned) had to first familiarize herself with the goals and the scope of the project. In the two weeks prior to the actual tracking of patients, the project coordinator developed a schedule for tracking each clinic based on knowledge of the routine days and times of clinic operations and planned clinic closures. The plan was to have the patients attending each clinic monitored twice and to selectively monitor clinics a third time, as time permitted. All staff involved in clinic operations required orientation to the project. Clinic physicians, nurses, secretaries, and staff outside the Department of Ambulatory Services, such as health records, phlebotomy, and other diagnostic assessment areas, were included. They received information about the project goals, the implementation plan, and instructions on how to complete the tracking form.

Crucial to the success of the project was the support of the chiefs of the departments of Surgery and Pediatrics, as well as the ongoing cooperation of the medical staff throughout the duration of the project. Time was spent initially to outline the goals of

Figure 14-1. Form Used to Track Service Time for One Clinic

Patient Name: _____ Hospital No.: _____

Clinic: _____ Date: _____

Registration Time: _____ Appointment Time: _____

Patient: Please hand this form to each hospital staff member you are seeing today.

Unit Clerk: **Patient:** (fill in and return)

Patient Check-in Time: _____ Patient Departure Time: _____

Physician	**Physician**	**Physician**
Time in: _____	Time in: _____	Time in: _____
Time out: _____	Time out: _____	Time out: _____
Seen by:	Seen by:	Seen by:
Resident _____	Resident _____	Resident _____
Staff Physician _____	Staff Physician _____	Staff Physician _____
Nurse	**Other**	**Other**
Time in: _____	Time in: _____	Time in: _____
Time out: _____	Time out: _____	Time out: _____
Activity: _____	Activity: _____	Activity: _____

Other Departments

X ray	**Bloodwork**	**Other**
Appointment: _____	Appointment: _____	Appointment: _____
Time in: _____	Time in: _____	Time in: _____
Time out: _____	Time out: _____	Time out: _____
Other: _____	**Other:** _____	**Other:** _____
Appointment: _____	Appointment: _____	Appointment: _____
Time in: _____	Time in: _____	Time in: _____
Time out: _____	Time out: _____	Time out: _____

---

the project and to explain the planned approach. Throughout the project, the medical coordinator remained highly visible and met formally and informally with physicians to ensure their ongoing support and cooperation.

For the initial patient tracking period, all clinics were tracked once over a two-week period. Clinics did not receive notification of the date of tracking prior to the actual day. Data entry and analysis of results were done in the following two-week period. For the second period of clinic tracking, clinics were tracked on alternate days of the week over a two- to four-week period in order to allow data entry and analysis to be done on the alternate days when tracking was not under way. This was a useful approach in that it allowed the project coordinator to discuss findings with the clinic staff while the events of the preceding day's clinic were still fresh in their minds.

On the day of clinic service time tracking, clinic secretaries initiated the tracking form for each patient by completing the patient and clinic demographic section of the form and recording the patient's time of arrival at the centralized registration desk, his or her scheduled clinic appointment time, and the time of the patient's actual check-in at the specific clinic registration desk. The tracking form was then placed at the front of the patient's health record. As the patient had contact with each member of the nursing, medical, or allied health staff or had a diagnostic procedure performed, the actual start and stop times of these encounters with the patient were recorded on the

175

Figure 14-2. Definitions of Terminology for a Time Tracking System

Diagnostic service: The time spent by the patient in the phlebotomy or diagnostic imaging area

Idle time: The cumulative time spent waiting as recorded on the tracking form

Nursing time: The time spent by the patient with a registered nurse or registered nursing assistant (does not include the time spent by the nurse discussing the patient with other members of the staff or the time spent in documentation of the contact)

Other: The time spent by the patient with a staff member of a nonmedical or nonnursing department, for example, occupational therapist, physiotherapist, dietitian, social worker, orthopedic technician, psychologist

Patient check-in time: The actual time the patient arrives at the designated clinic reception desk

Physician time: The time spent by the patient with a medical student, resident, fellow, or staff physician (does not include the time spent by the physician discussing the patient with other members of the staff or the time spent in documentation of the contact)

Registration time: The actual time of registration at the outpatient department registration desk, as recorded on the registration form

Time to first contact: The time spent from check-in at the clinic reception desk until initial contact with a physician or nurse

Total service time: The time from check-in at the clinic to departure from the clinic or area of last testing or service

tracking form. Patients were instructed to return the form to the specific clinic registration desk at the end of the day so that the clinic secretary could record their time of departure. Tracking forms were retained by the clinic secretary for return to the project coordinator at the end of the clinic day. Additionally, copies of the clinic appointment list for the day, and a list of the unscheduled patients who were seen, were provided to the project coordinator.

□ Data Analysis

Determination of patients' clinic service times was done after the data contained on the clinic tracking form were entered into the computer. For each clinic monitored, a clinic report was generated (see figure 14-3). Information contained in the report included the summary of the clinic demographics, including the number of patients booked, the number of patients seen by a clinic provider, and the number of patients tracked by the monitoring system. Patient arrival times were reported, showing a breakdown of early, on-time, and late arrivals as measured against the patients' scheduled appointment times. The final section contained in the clinic report was a time analysis (in minutes) of the various amounts of time that patients in the clinic spent with providers, with other care givers, or waiting for service (idle time).

The report shows that of the 30 patients tracked, all saw physicians; and on average, each spent 13 minutes with his or her physician. The least amount of time a patient spent with the physician was 4 minutes, and the maximum was 45 minutes. The average amount of idle time spent by the patients was 81 minutes, with a minimum of 15 and a maximum of 249 minutes. The average total service time that a patient experienced during the visit to this particular clinic (Clinic 3413) on this particular day (January 23, 1990) was 106 minutes. The average length of time between the patients' arrival and first contact with a physician, a nurse, or other direct care giver was 55 minutes.

Figure 14-4 (p. 178) shows another report generated by the system. For the same clinic as noted above (Clinic 3413), the data were sorted by patient arrival time so that each of the 30 patients was represented on the graph from first to last arrival. This

Figure 14-3. Report of Service Time Tracking for One Clinic

Clinic report for: 3413   Date: 01/23/90   Time: 800

Clinic information:

Appointments booked	47
Arrivals not on list	8
Appointments as no-shows	8
Number of appointments seen	47
Number of appointments tracked	30

Arrivals	Number	Average minutes
Early	10	18
On time	0	
Late	15	20

Time analysis (minutes)

	Number	Average	Minimum	Maximum	Total
Physicians	30	13	4	45	399
Nurses	17	3	1	33	56
Bloodwork	0	0	0	0	0
X ray	13	15	2	31	195
Other services	5	22	0	45	110
Idle time		81	15	249	
Total service time		106	28	310	
First contact		55	0	163	

graphical representation was used to determine the flow of patients through a clinic. Once the data for each clinic associated with a particular clinical division were entered into the computer and analyzed, summary reports of clinic operations for each clinical division were generated.

☐ Project Findings

The ambulatory care clinic services of the 26 clinical divisions within the departments of Pediatrics and Surgery at The Hospital for Sick Children were included in the project. In total, 142 clinics were monitored, and the clinic service times of 1,919 patients were analyzed. This number represented an 83 percent return rate. In the majority of clinics included in the project, the mean and the median service times were similar. In many of these clinics, this related to the amount of time required to assess and treat patients with complex illness and accommodate their families. However, data analysis showed that the components of the total service times varied among the clinics as a result of a number of factors, including patient complexity and clinic volumes.

Figure 14-5 shows a summary of the patient service times (in minutes) for a sample of patients attending the medical specialty clinics. For example, for the clinical division of cardiology, 70 patients were tracked and, on average, their total service time was 100 minutes. The median for the cardiology clinics was 94 minutes, indicating that times for half of the 70 patients tracked fell below 94 minutes and half of them had values greater than 94 minutes. The range of the total service time was as low as 29 minutes and as high as 204 minutes, which meant that at least one patient spent 3.4 hours at the hospital for his or her ambulatory care clinic visit.

Figure 14-4. Graph Showing Data by Patient Arrival Time for One Morning Clinic

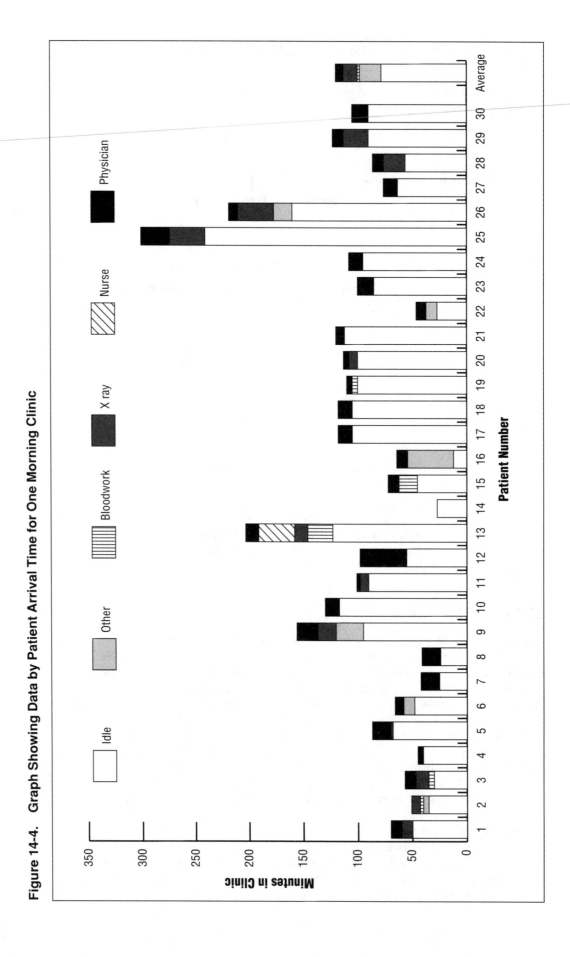

Figure 14-5. Summary of Patient Service Times (in Minutes)

Medical Specialties, Clinical Division	Number of Patients	Component	Mean	Median	Range
Adolescent Medicine	48	Total service	64	63	20–145
		Idle	17	10	0–85
		Idle as percentage of total service time	26	16	
		Time to first contact	11	10	0–80
		Physician	43	28	0–90
		Nurse	47	0	0–140
		Diagnostic services	2	0	0–4
		Other	50	0	0–95
Cardiology	70	Total service	100	94	29–204
		Idle	55	47	0–132
		Idle as percentage of total service time	55	50	
		Time to first contact	15	6	0–86
		Physician	23	20	0–114
		Nurse	9	7	0–29
		Diagnostic services	15	0	0–58
		Other	10	5	0–70
Chest	108	Total service	78	72	12–190
		Idle	43	41	5–127
		Idle as percentage of total service time	55	57	
		Time to first contact	13	10	0–75
		Physician	22	17	2–75
		Nurse	7	5	0–25
		Diagnostic services	19	0	0–50
		Other	17	0	0–45
Clinical Genetics	17	Total service	95	105	45–207
		Idle	45	30	0–132
		Idle as percentage of total service time	47	29	
		Time to first contact	11	10	0–30
		Physician	22	15	0–30
		Nurse	19	10	2–40
		Diagnostic services	6	0	0–10
		Other	20	30	0–85
Clinical Nutrition	18	Total service	70	66	35–118
		Idle	29	21	5–99
		Idle as percentage of total service time	41	32	
		Time to first contact	10	7	0–33
		Physician	35	30	14–76
		Nurse	6	5	0–10
		Diagnostic services	1	0	0–2
		Other	0	0	0

Figure 14-6 shows the mean or average values for each component of total service time by geographical areas. At The Hospital for Sick Children, the clinics operated by the clinical division of General Pediatrics were included in the general medical clinics geographical area, all of the Department of Pediatrics medical specialty clinics were incorporated into the medical specialties numbers, and the surgical area included the surgical divisions. The average total service times were similar in the three geographical

Figure 14-6. Graph Showing Mean Values for Total Service Times, by Geographical Area

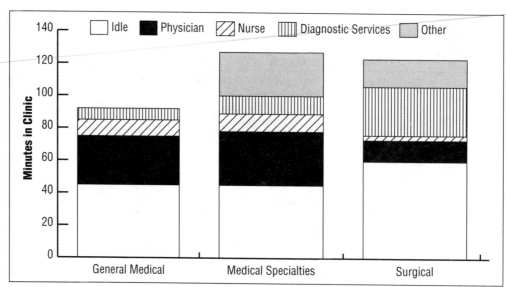

areas at 80–87 minutes. This is not actually represented on the graph, as the graph represents the average time for each service component separately, and the sum of the component averages is not the same as the average total service time.

The proportion of idle time is indicated by the black band at the base of each of the three bar graphs. The graph shows that the proportion of idle time was greatest in the surgical clinics (58 minutes). This represented 73 percent of the mean total service time for the surgical clinics. The least amount of idle time was evident in the general medical and medical specialty clinics, and these times are shown on the graph as 44 minutes. These numbers represented 44 percent of the average total service time for patients included in the general medical subset and almost one-third of the total service time for patients included in the medical specialty subset. The physician and nurse components of total service time were shortest in the surgical clinics and were greatest in the general medical clinics. In the surgical clinics, for instance, the amount of physician and nursing time was about 12 minutes total, compared with the general medical/medical specialty clinics, where the physician and nursing times were much greater. Nursing time was felt to be underrepresented in this study because some of the clinics included in the sample did not have an assigned nurse; and in many clinics, when the physician and the nurse saw the patient simultaneously, only the physician time was recorded.

The other main difference to be seen on the graph is the general medical clinics' lack of time associated with the use of "other" services, which included services provided by allied health and ancillary services. Both the medical specialty and surgical clinics had times associated with referrals to these areas included in their average total service times.

Figure 14-7 shows the median values for the total service times by each of the three geographical areas. The median total service times were similar in all areas and ranged between 69 and 73 minutes. This means that half of the patients tracked had total service times of less than 69–73 minutes and half the patients had total service times of more than 69–73 minutes. This graph shows variability among the components of total service time similar to that shown in figure 14-6.

For the patients included in the project, the total service time ranged from as short as three minutes to as long as five hours. Idle time showed a similar variability, ranging from no idle time to 4.5 hours. The longest idle times occurred in some of the surgical

Figure 14-7. Graph Showing Median Values for Total Service Times, by Geographical Area

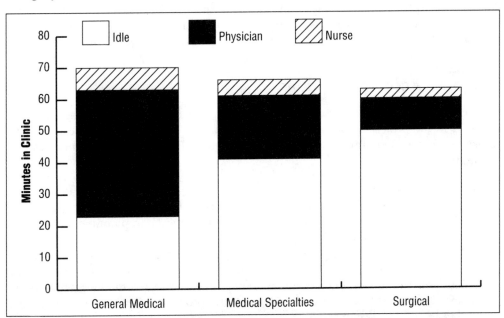

and medical specialty clinics. Analysis of this idle time showed that, in general, idle time accumulated in small amounts throughout the patient's clinic visit, rather than all at once at the beginning of the appointment. It was found, for example, that patients waited from the time they checked in with the clinic secretary until their first contact with the clinic nurse; next, they waited to have a diagnostic test done or to see the physician. Before leaving the hospital after their consultation with the physician, patients may also have experienced another short wait for the scheduling of follow-up appointments.

Other factors that were incorporated in the idle-time component of the total service time included the following:

- Consultation among professional staff about specific patients
- Delays waiting for the retrieval of health records, X rays, or diagnostic test results
- Time spent by the patient traveling between diagnostic and assessment areas within the ambulatory care setting
- Time spent waiting for the analysis and interpretation of diagnostic tests or procedures to be reported

Additional observations related to the factors contributing to idle time showed that at The Hospital for Sick Children, diagnostic testing of ambulatory care patients tended to be done in the morning. As a result, patients with morning appointments were able to complete their clinic visit, including their diagnostic testings, within the morning period. Patients who had afternoon clinic appointments generally had longer service times because they completed the diagnostic tests or procedures in the morning and then had to wait until the afternoon to be seen in the clinic.

On the basis of an analysis of the general and clinic-specific findings, a number of consistent issues were identified. First, the booking systems for many of the ambulatory care clinics were designed to facilitate the operation of the clinic, rather than minimize idle times and total service times for patients. Second, the demand was high for clinic appointments, particularly for surgical ones, resulting in large patient volumes being seen in clinics. Third, delays occurred in all the clinic areas, and many of them were unavoidable due to the complexity of the patient's condition. However, in many cases the patient and the family arrived unprepared for these waiting periods. In a pediatric setting where there are concerns about small children and the care of other family members who may remain at home, this created problems for the families.

□ Project Recommendations

Specific recommendations were generated for each of the 26 clinical divisions that were included in the project. In addition, general recommendations were proposed for all clinic areas in the Department of Ambulatory Services. These recommendations can be summarized as follows:

- All appointment systems should be reviewed regularly to ensure that bookings are planned to optimize the care and the service for the patient and the family. The ease of clinic operation is obviously a consideration in planning, but patient care should be the priority.
- The possibility of preappointment mailing or distribution of clinic information should be considered in order to adequately prepare patients and families for the clinic experience. The possibility of idle time as well as strategies for handling this time should be included in this information. For example, in a pediatric setting, it is important to give parents guidance concerning appropriate toys and nutritional snacks to bring with them.
- A centralized diagnostic service should be established to assist in the coordination of booking appointments for diagnostic services. During planning of this service, consideration should be given to reserving times for or giving priority to diagnostic appointments that would more closely coincide with morning and afternoon clinic appointments.
- Clinic staff should encourage the staff, the providers, and the patients to arrive on time because early as well as late arrivals tend to disrupt the flow of patients through the various clinics.
- The ambulatory care clinic management team, together with the nursing staff, should examine the nursing component of total service time. This would be particularly relevant for the surgical clinics. Enhancing the role of the nurse in areas such as patient assessment, teaching, and counseling would optimize patient care and would further help to reduce the amount of idle time patients experience.
- Physicians, in particular surgeons, should be careful in scheduling their meetings and operating room times in order to preserve sufficient time to see clinic patients.
- The staff of the Department of Ambulatory Services should ensure the accuracy of the typed appointment list to help eliminate avoidable delays in retrieving health records and X rays. This recommendation mainly involved the clerical staff of the clinic, but it also included the medical staff, who need to inform clinic secretaries of last-minute or other add-on patients.
- Consideration may need to be given to the addition of evening or extended hours of clinic operations, particularly in the case of clinics where there is a high demand for appointments.

□ Lessons Learned

The first questions that come to mind in concluding such a project and evaluating future steps are: What lessons were learned? and Should a project of this type be done again? Following are some of the lessons learned:

- Adopting a pragmatic approach when designing and fine-tuning the system allowed for development of a system that was workable in a large and complex setting.
- Having the involvement and commitment of key physician leaders for the duration of the project was instrumental to its success.
- The selection of a clinic nurse as project coordinator was important. The nurse was well known to physicians and clinic staff alike and she was able to communicate easily with both groups.
- It was also important to have a full-time coordinator in order to keep the various components on track and to complete the project within the projected time frame.
- Given the scale of ambulatory care clinic operations at the Hospital and the complexity of the project, project management skills and technical support in the form of custom-designed software, a computer, and a printer were essential for data analysis and report writing.

☐ Project Outcomes

Overall, the project achieved a successful outcome, and the results were tangible for patients, for providers, and for management. There was heightened awareness within the hospital about clinic operations and, more specifically, patient and family service times. This resulted from ongoing and final project reporting to senior management, physician groups, and each of the clinical divisions. A system for objectively measuring clinic service times was developed, tested, and refined for use. Reporting findings and recommendations to clinical division heads together with their clinic nurses and secretaries at joint meetings was extremely useful. It provided an opportunity for increased communication among all levels of the staff involved in specific clinics, and it provided them with an opportunity—often for the first time—to review clinic operations and to establish common goals and approaches for resolution of any issues. Patients and families perceived that something was being done. Throughout the project, they were cooperative and supportive. Objective data were obtained as a result of the implementation of the system, and providers and clinic management teams had an opportunity to review the recommendations, agree to them, and implement them.

The centralized diagnostic booking service was also initiated as a result of this project. Clinic staff made revisions to the patient scheduling practices, and although all is not perfect, there has been a hospitalwide perception of improvement. This is supported by the fact that the Hospital president no longer receives daily or weekly letters or calls of complaint from patients or families.

A year later, the Hospital is in the process of remonitoring the service times in selected clinics. Although the data analysis is incomplete as of this writing, the initial impression is that the total service times and the amount of idle time that patients experience have been reduced. This remonitoring of times in selected clinics is being done by the nurses associated with each clinic, with assistance from the project coordinator. This has been useful in that there is now a pool of expertise for monitoring clinic service times within the ambulatory care setting.

As a next step, the hospital plans to remonitor the service times in all of the clinical divisions in the upcoming year to ensure that the desired results were achieved and, more important, were maintained. The intention is to report the results as before, because this provided clinic staff and physicians with an opportunity for communication and for review of their progress.

☐ Conclusion

It is generally agreed that the measurement of quality in ambulatory care services must include the component of patient satisfaction. Therefore, the challenge faced by

183

ambulatory care providers is to develop patient satisfaction surveys that yield meaningful information from which improvement decisions can be made.

The focused patient satisfaction project at The Hospital for Sick Children is a good example of how this challenge can be met through careful survey design, involvement of ambulatory care staff in all phases of the project, and establishment of information management systems that enhance the analysis of the survey results. Careful planning in the survey design and implementation phases was critical to the success of the project. Sharing the project goals with each ambulatory care provider group and the medical director enhanced their understanding of the survey and helped garner their cooperation in what could have been viewed as a burdensome data collection task. And, of course, computer support helped to augment the reporting and analysis of the survey results.

The focused patient satisfaction survey was a great success. It achieved the clinic's quality measurement objectives by providing valuable information about the root causes of patient service time delays—information that could be used to target improvements in the processes that were contributing to those delays.

Section Eight

Ambulatory Care Quality Measurement Programs That Compare Providers

The quality of ambulatory care services must meet professionally recognized standards on both an individual-case basis and in the aggregate. The ideal quality measurement process incorporates the use of comparative data derived from the experience of other organizations or individuals. When performance is found to differ from that of other groups, the reasons for that difference should be investigated and offer an opportunity for performance enhancement. Comparative data also offer a yardstick for continuous improvement. An ambulatory care provider that consistently meets its internal quality expectations might well ask, "Could we do even better, and if so, how?"

The authors in this section describe two comprehensive projects that yield comparative quality information for ambulatory care providers. Chapter 15 describes an office practice liability control project initiated at the state level and now being offered nationally to physicians in private practice. Chapter 16 describes a quality review project that allows primary care physicians to compare their clinical and office system performance to that of others.

Chapter 15

Office-Based Risk Assessment Program

Paul Frisch, J.D.

U p to one-third of liability claims against physicians are tied to something that happened in the medical office. To help physicians address the nonclinical aspects of office practice that are known to play a role in malpractice suits, the integrated nonclinical office practice assessment and quality improvement program (PA/QI) was developed by a coalition of medical organizations. This is the first comprehensive, data-based risk management program created for the ambulatory care setting.

The Oregon Medical Association (OMA) developed and tested the PA/QI program in collaboration with the American Medical Association/Specialty Society Medical Liability Project (AMA/SSMLP). The AMA/SSMLP is a coalition of more than 30 national medical specialty societies, the AMA, and the Council of Medical Specialty Societies formed for the purpose of coordinating the professional liability activities of organized medicine. Oregon is an ideal laboratory for the development of a program such as PA/QI. The OMA has for many years been a leader in the field of loss-prevention education, creating an ongoing series of highly effective and innovative loss-prevention education programs for its 5,000 member physicians.[1]

In April 1991, based on the preliminary results of Oregon's experience with PA/QI, the patient safety/risk management subcommittee of the AMA/SSMLP embarked on the ambitious task of adapting PA/QI to offer it nationally. Currently the AMA/SSMLP is working with several state medical associations and liability insurers in a countrywide demonstration project.

The OMA developed its PA/QI prototype for primary care physicians. There were two reasons for this. First, primary care physicians are the largest grouping of specialties insured under OMA's physician protection program. Second, OMA has documented a shift in claim frequency away from the hospital and into the ambulatory care setting. Not only have the number of outpatient procedures increased, but the plaintiffs' bar

This chapter is copyrighted by Paul Frisch and the American Medical Association, 1992. The author would like to thank Charlotte Miller for her assistance in the writing of this chapter. Ms. Miller is a staff associate in the Department of Professional Liability and Insurance, Health Law Division, of the American Medical Association, Chicago, and program director of the Practice Assessment/Quality Improvement Program for the AMA/Specialty Society Medical Liability Project.

has placed renewed emphasis on failure-to-diagnose claims. Most of the claims alleging a failure to diagnose have originated in the medical office setting.

Nineteen Oregon physicians participated in the PA/QI pilot program in 1990. During 1991, an additional 52 physicians participated.

☐ Components of the PA/QI Process

The PA/QI program updates and unites three methods of loss-prevention education that are usually presented separately: a self-assessment survey of nonclinical office practice activities, a home-study course, and on-site visitation. By fully integrating these three components, PA/QI becomes more than the sum of its parts. A specialty-specific, data-based educational activity, PA/QI can monitor and evaluate its participants' ongoing experience to demonstrate longitudinally that changes in nonclinical office practice systems, procedures, and behaviors reduce both the frequency and severity of malpractice claims.

Self-Assessment Survey

The PA/QI self-assessment survey (SAS) consists of 103 questions addressing nonclinical aspects of office practice (see figure 15-1). To assist in analyzing the results, participants also provide demographic data about their specialty, age, sex, practice type, number of physicians in their office, geographical location and other information, including malpractice claims history.

The PA/QI survey shown in figure 15-1 is a modification of the one used in OMA's pilot project. The AMA/SSMLP added or deleted some questions and reworded most of the others. In addition, AMA/SSMLP expanded the amount of demographic data collected by the survey questionnaire. This was done to ensure collection of a uniform demographic data set without relying on tie-ins to outside data bases, which may not be possible to do for all PA/QI participants nationwide.

In Oregon, demographic data concerning specialty, age, and sex of participants are obtained by linking the SAS data base to OMA's membership data base. Each participant's OMA identification number is cross-referenced in each of the PA/QI's data bases. Thus, most demographic data elements are supplied automatically.

A count of all reported malpractice claims and the amount of any settlements and awards are obtained by linking the same identification number to an OMA data base of more than 4,200 Oregon malpractice claims dating back to 1972. Finally, if a participant's office personnel have completed a similar SAS medical office staff questionnaire, those data are available from a separate data base of more than 1,000 responses. By the end of 1991, a total of some 2,000 physician surveys and some 1,500 office personnel surveys had been completed and processed.

The PA/QI self-assessment survey has two distinct but equally important functions. The first is to deliver an educational message. By completing the SAS, participants have the opportunity to review and reflect on a broad spectrum of nonclinical risk management objectives related to office practice. The act of completing the survey prompts many physicians to initiate needed practice and behavior changes that they may previously have been unaware of, overlooked, or ignored. The educational message is subsequently reinforced when each participant receives an individual assessment report (figure 15-2, p. 194). This report shows the participants how they stack up against not only their peers but all other survey participants as well. By collecting detailed demographic information, PA/QI can create a participant's "peer group" with great precision. This gives the PA/QI program enhanced credibility with participants, because their peer group profile closely matches their own demographic and practice characteristics.

Figure 15-1. Self-Assessment Survey: Medical Office Practice

(Score one point for each "No" answer)

A. HOW WELL DOES MY OFFICE REPRESENT ME? (THE PATIENT'S EYE VIEW)

29. I keep office hours which enable me to see all scheduled patients.

____Yes   ____No   ____n/a

30. My patients perceive the waiting/reception area as pleasant.

____Yes   ____No   ____n/a

31. There are sufficient chairs in the waiting room.

____Yes   ____No   ____n/a

32. I make up-to-date, patient-related medical literature available to my patients.

____Yes   ____No   ____n/a

33. My receptionist makes a good impression on the telephone.

____Yes   ____No   ____n/a

34. Patients cannot hear telephone conversations at the front desk while in the waiting room.

____Yes   ____No   ____n/a

35. Patients in the waiting room cannot overhear personal conversations between staff members.

____Yes   ____No   ____n/a

36. Patients are notified if I am running behind in seeing patients.

____Yes   ____No   ____n/a

Section Total _____

B. APPOINTMENTS/TERMINATION

37. I book only the number of appointments I can properly handle.

____Yes   ____No   ____n/a

38. On average, my patients with an appointment spend less than 30 minutes in the waiting room.

____Yes   ____No   ____n/a

39. On average, it take my patients less than two weeks to get an appointment.

____Yes   ____No   ____n/a

40. I have an established procedure for my staff to follow up on missed appointments.

____Yes   ____No   ____n/a

41. The results of the follow-up on missed appointments are entered in a record and/or posted in the patient's chart.

____Yes   ____No   ____n/a

42. I give the patient my reasons for termination of the doctor-patient relationship in writing.

____Yes   ____No   ____n/a

Section Total _____

C. DO MY PATIENTS AND I GET OFF TO A GOOD PROFESSIONAL START?

43. I, or someone else in my office, discusses fees and other charges with my patients.

____Yes   ____No   ____n/a

44. I, or someone else in my office, discusses methods of payment with my patients.

____Yes   ____No   ____n/a

45. If I am practicing with one or more physicians in the same specialty, the patient has an option as to who will treat him/her.

____Yes   ____No   ____n/a

46. New patient history is taken by me or by another qualified person in my office.

____Yes   ____No   ____n/a

47. Patients are specifically asked about allergies, sensitivities, bad results, etc., and the answers are then entered in their charts.

____Yes   ____No   ____n/a

(continued on next page)

Second, the survey serves an invaluable data-gathering function. Periodic analysis of aggregate SAS data allows tailored risk management messages to be delivered to precisely crafted audiences. When loss data suggest there is a correlation with certain practice or behavior patterns reflected in the SAS, an organization can use PA/QI data to efficiently and economically target its audience and then focus its resources on a particular specialty, office practice type, age range, geographical area, or physician grouping with prior claims to enhance the impact of its messages. An example of Oregon SAS data appears in figure 15-3 (p. 195).

Periodic re-surveys make it possible to measure the extent to which PA/QI and related risk management efforts have positively influenced the behavior of physicians

Figure 15-1. (Continued)

48. I require a complete physical exam for all new patients.

___Yes ___No ___n/a

49. Most patients feel that I have pleasant and private examining rooms.

___Yes ___No ___n/a

Section Total _____

D. ARE MY PATIENTS AND I PROTECTED BY MY OFFICE PROCEDURES?
---

50. Certain lab tests, if urgent, are performed in-office.

___Yes ___No ___n/a

51. An outside lab is used whenever appropriate.

___Yes ___No ___n/a

52. There is an established procedure for informing the patient of all office and outside lab results.

___Yes ___No ___n/a

53. I have a fail-safe follow-up system for a patient who is referred for diagnostic testing.

___Yes ___No ___n/a

54. I review all incoming medical lab and consultant reports before they are placed into the patient's chart.

___Yes ___No ___n/a

55. Injections are only administered by me or other qualified persons.

___Yes ___No ___n/a

56. I have an efficient, well-run patient reminder system for yearly examinations.

___Yes ___No ___n/a

57. I am qualified by training to cover for all physicians with whom I share call.

___Yes ___No ___n/a

58. I request all the necessary records when I see a patient in consultation.

___Yes ___No ___n/a

59. I have an established follow-up system when I refer a patient to a consultant.

___Yes ___No ___n/a

60. The physicians who cover for me are qualified by training to do so.

___Yes ___No ___n/a

61. Patients are told in advance who is covering.

___Yes ___No ___n/a

62. I have an after-hours answering service.

___Yes ___No ___n/a

63. Calls are answered by a person, not an electronic device.

___Yes ___No ___n/a

64. X-rays/ultrasound, if performed in the office, are carried out by a qualified person.

___Yes ___No ___n/a

65. My office equipment (X-ray, ultrasound, etc.) is checked as required.

___Yes ___No ___n/a

66. ECG's performed in the office are taken by a trained person and read by a qualified person.

___Yes ___No ___n/a

67. If a patient refuses to follow my instructions, I have a set protocol for dealing with the non-compliance problem.

___Yes ___No ___n/a

68. If a patient of the opposite sex is having an examination involving private parts, a member of my staff who is the same sex as the patient is always present.

___Yes ___No ___n/a

Section Total _____

E. IS MY DRUG CONTROL ADEQUATE?
---

69. Prescription pads are kept out of sight of patients.

___Yes ___No ___n/a

and their office personnel. Furthermore, it is hoped that PA/QI data will make a valuable contribution to research examining the utility of risk management practices in improving patient care and preventing liability claims.

Home-Study Course

The home-study course consists of a workbook containing five Physician Practice Reviews, each describing a hypothetical physician and his or her medical malpractice claims. Actual claims, disguised to protect confidentiality, are used. Participants review the hypothetical physicians' practice and behavior patterns as well as their claims in an effort to determine what makes the hypothetical physicians vulnerable to liability

Figure 15-1. (Continued)

70. Syringes are kept out of sight.

_____Yes   _____No   _____n/a

71. Drugs are kept out of sight.

_____Yes   _____No   _____n/a

72. Locked.

_____Yes   _____No   _____n/a

73. Purged.

_____Yes   _____No   _____n/a

74. Different drugs are kept in separate locations.

_____Yes   _____No   _____n/a

75. Different drugs are kept in different sized and colored containers.

_____Yes   _____No   _____n/a

76. An adequate drug record is kept of all narcotic drugs.

_____Yes   _____No   _____n/a

Section Total _____

F. DO MY BILLING AND COLLECTION PROCEDURES UNNECESSARILY ANTAGONIZE SOME PATIENTS OR GIVE THEM REASON TO BE RESENTFUL?

77. I always review the patient's chart before initiating aggressive collection procedures.

_____Yes   _____No   _____n/a

78. Aggressive collection is not pursued without my approval.

_____Yes   _____No   _____n/a

79. If and when a collection agency is used, the agency's efforts are monitored and suits are not allowed without my express permission.

_____Yes   _____No   _____n/a

80. If a patient questions my professional fees, I insist on being informed.

_____Yes   _____No   _____n/a

81. If I terminate treatment of a patient who has an overdue account, I do so in writing, by certified mail, return receipt requested, provide a grace period and offer to help locate other professional health care.

_____Yes   _____No   _____n/a

Section Total _____

G. WHEN MY PATIENT CALLS, HOW IS IT HANDLED?

82. There are a sufficient number of telephone lines into my office.

_____Yes   _____No   _____n/a

83. The staff waits for the patient's permission before placing the patient on hold.

_____Yes   _____No   _____n/a

84. The average time a patient is on hold is less than 2 minutes.

_____Yes   _____No   _____n/a

85. My receptionist, when screening calls, is careful not to build a barrier between me and my patient.

_____Yes   _____No   _____n/a

86. I accept calls when requested to do so by my staff.

_____Yes   _____No   _____n/a

87. My staff has been instructed not to renew prescriptions without my approval.

_____Yes   _____No   _____n/a

Section Total _____

H. DO THE MEDICAL RECORDS IN MY OFFICE PROTECT MY PATIENT AND ME IF A MEDICAL PROBLEM DEVELOPS?

88. I chart the reason for the patient's visit, including all complaints.

_____Yes   _____No   _____n/a

(continued on next page)

claims. The objective is to sensitize participants to these areas of vulnerability in a nonthreatening way, focusing first on hypothetical colleagues and then asking the participant to assess whether any of these problems are or could be present in his or her own practice.

The Physician Practice Reviews are specialty-specific. A primary care version for family physicians, internists, and pediatricians was developed first. Versions for other specialties are under development and will become available beginning in late 1992.

In Oregon, videotaped vignettes are provided that depict the five hypothetical physicians and show nonverbal behaviors and interactions with patients and colleagues that may play a role in precipitating malpractice claims. Two reference pieces help

Figure 15-1. (Continued)

89. I chart patient's history, including past medical treatments, current medications, drug allergies, family history, etc.

____Yes   ____No   ____n/a

90. My patients fill out a questionnaire on their current complaints and previous history.

____Yes   ____No   ____n/a

91. If yes, I document my review and follow-up on the questionnaire.

____Yes   ____No   ____n/a

92. Also, I document my investigation of question marks and blank spaces left on the questionnaire.

____Yes   ____No   ____n/a

93. I chart all my physical findings.

____Yes   ____No   ____n/a

94. I chart negative findings.

____Yes   ____No   ____n/a

95. I diagram size and location of suspicious lumps and lesions.

____Yes   ____No   ____n/a

96. If yes, my patients sign or initial these diagrams.

____Yes   ____No   ____n/a

Section Total _____

I. DIAGNOSIS

97. I chart the data used to support my diagnostic impressions.

____Yes   ____No   ____n/a

98. I review and initial all path, lab and X-ray reports.

____Yes   ____No   ____n/a

99. I review available previous medical reports and then chart appropriate data.

____Yes   ____No   ____n/a

100. I chart discussions with other providers that lead to the diagnosis.

____Yes   ____No   ____n/a

Section Total _____

J. TREATMENT

101. I outline a treatment plan that is supported by the findings in the workup and diagnosis.

____Yes   ____No   ____n/a

102. I chart obtaining the patient's informed consent.

____Yes   ____No   ____n/a

103. When appropriate, I chart the patient's informed refusal.

____Yes   ____No   ____n/a

104. I chart all instructions to the patient, including follow-up requirements.

____Yes   ____No   ____n/a

Section Total _____

K. FOLLOW-UP

105. I chart who is responsible for follow-up, me or the patient.

____Yes   ____No   ____n/a

106. I chart recommendations for referral to outside care or follow-up.

____Yes   ____No   ____n/a

107. I chart discussions with other providers about patient care.

____Yes   ____No   ____n/a

108. I chart consideration of previous findings in follow-up.

____Yes   ____No   ____n/a

109. I chart unchanged abnormal findings.

____Yes   ____No   ____n/a

participants do the Physician Practice Review exercises: AMA/SSMLP's *Risk Management Principles & Commentaries for the Medical Office;* and "Lessons From Oregon's RAMP Program," an article listing practice patterns and behaviors that OMA found to be associated with physicians who have had multiple claims filed against them. (RAMP is the acronym for OMA's Risk Assessment and Management Program.)

On-Site Visitation

The third part of the integrated PA/QI process is an on-site visit to the participant's office. A frequent underwriting tool of malpractice insurers, the office visit in the PA/

Figure 15-1. (Continued)

110. I chart my review of subsequent lab/X-ray reports.

____Yes   ____No   ____n/a

111. I chart patient compliance or non-compliance with recommendations.

____Yes   ____No   ____n/a

Section Total _____

L. OFFICE CHARTING PROCEDURES

112. Missed/canceled appointments (reason included, if known) are noted on the patient's chart.

____Yes   ____No   ____n/a

113. All telephone conversations (physician and staff) regarding patient care are noted on the chart.

____Yes   ____No   ____n/a

114. All drug allergies are noted prominently on the chart.

____Yes   ____No   ____n/a

115. All lab/X-ray reports are seen and initialed by me before placement in the chart.

____Yes   ____No   ____n/a

116. Signed, dated authorizations are obtained and placed in the chart before copies of the chart are released.

____Yes   ____No   ____n/a

117. It is noted on the chart where the copy is being sent.

____Yes   ____No   ____n/a

118. My authorization is required before records can be released.

____Yes   ____No   ____n/a

119. There is a stated procedure for termination of care that is followed in my office.

____Yes   ____No   ____n/a

Section Total _____

M. CHARTING HABITS

120. Chart notes are readable.

____Yes   ____No   ____n/a

121. All chart entries are dated.

____Yes   ____No   ____n/a

122. Corrections and additions to the chart are entered chronologically, dated and signed.

____Yes   ____No   ____n/a

123. In my absence, a colleague using information from the medical chart could provide my patient with immediate and appropriate care.

____Yes   ____No   ____n/a

Section Total _____

QI model is conducted for different reasons. It is believed that changes that occur by choice rather than by directive are more likely to become a permanent part of a physician's practice.

For the national PA/QI demonstration project, pilot sites are being relied upon to develop the office visit component in accord with local circumstances. Although this may result in variations in certain particulars (for example, whether a physician or other trained person performs the chart review), all PA/QI visits are expected to accomplish the same goals of evaluating and reinforcing the effectiveness of the risk management messages introduced in Parts One and Two of the program.

During the on-site phase of the PA/QI process in Oregon, practice surveyors use the self-assessment surveys and the home-study course evaluations to identify areas of

Figure 15-2. Excerpt from Individual Assessment Report

Nonclinical Office Practice Matters.Needing Attention

Physician's number	790		
Specialty	Internist		
Office type	Single		
Number of claims	4		
Total indemnity paid	$136,000.00		

	Your Response	Your Specialty		All Surveys	
	Number of Yes Responses	Total Responses	Total Matching Your Response	Total Responses	Total Matching Your Response
#30: Patients hear telephone conversations while in waiting room	150	70	47%	690	299 43%
#38: Patients with appointments wait no more than 30 minutes	153	12	8%	693	57 8%
#56: There is no patient reminder system for yearly examinations	150	82	55%	608	312 51%
#79: Collection agency efforts are not monitored	143	30	21%	673	144 21%
#87: Staff renews prescriptions without physician approval	155	16	10%	661	42 6%
#113: Telephone calls are not charted	155	48	31%	687	228 33%

concern. This enables them to focus the limited time and financial resources of the program on relevant nonclinical risk management difficulties. Randomly selected office charts are reviewed by a physician. A report concerning their adequacy is generated and shared with each participant. Key staff in the participating physician's office complete an SAS before the surveyor's visit. Their individual assessment reports are an important mechanism for verifying the accuracy of the physician's own perceptions about the practice and behavior patterns of a particular office.

Surveyors spend approximately two and one-half hours in each office interviewing both physicians and key staff. An officewide "wrap-up" session is held at the visit's close to communicate the findings of the review and to discuss strategies for achieving agreed-on practice changes. In Oregon, yearly follow-up visits are planned. Additionally, each participant's future malpractice claims are tracked in OMA's data base. A program "tags" subsequent claims, if any, and alerts OMA staff, which can then investigate to determine whether and how any of the behaviors and practice patterns in the PA/QI process affected the claim.

☐ Premises Underlying the PA/QI Effort

Development of the PA/QI program was guided by three tenets. First, lasting changes in behavior result from personal motivation, not externally applied mandates (as already noted). The PA/QI program relies on the professionals' internal commitment to quality

Figure 15-3. Excerpt from Targeted Analysis Report

Selected Questions, Comparison by Selected Group

Question #40: There is no procedure for staff follow-up on appointments.

Grouping	Responses	Number of No's	Percent
All Surveys by Specialty:	1,419	459	32
Anesthesiology	27	5	19
Diagnostic Radiology	29	12	41
Emergency Medicine	3	1	33
Family Practice	221	103	47
General Practice	41	17	41
Internal Medicine	292	106	36
Neurosurgery	18	3	17
Obstetrics/Gynecology	89	14	16
Ophthalmology	108	21	19
Orthopedic Surgery	27	8	30
Pathology	17	2	12
Pediatrics	80	27	34
Radiology	51	18	35
Surgery	91	21	23
Therapeutic Radiology	3		
Thoracic Surgery	2		
Vascular Surgery	7	1	14

Question #41: Results of follow-up on missed appointments not entered in chart.

Grouping	Responses	Number of No's	Percent
All Surveys by Specialty:	1,377	366	27
Anesthesiology	27	4	15
Diagnostic Radiology	26	19	73
Emergency Medicine	2		
Family Practice	217	67	31
General Practice	40	12	30
Internal Medicine	284	88	31
Neurosurgery	17	3	18
Obstetrics/Gynecology	89	9	10
Ophthalmology	102	13	13
Orthopedic Surgery	27	10	37
Pathology	13	3	23
Pediatrics	77	21	27
Radiology	47	24	51
Surgery	89	12	13
Therapeutic Radiology	3	1	33
Thoracic Surgery	2		
Vascular Surgery	7		

rather than their fear of retribution. Second, reasonable suggestions for minimizing liability risk must be offered to physicians. The risk management recommendations presented in the PA/QI program, gleaned from the experience of other physicians, are easily incorporated into a physician's everyday practice. Third, the risk-prevention program must have a specialty-specific component. Whereas many (if not most) medical office risk management issues are not specialty-specific, it is important to recognize that specialty differences do exist, and also, that the most effective learning experience is one that mirrors each participant's specialty as much as possible.

Aspiration, Not Fear, Promotes Successful Quality Improvement

According to Berwick, who has long and successfully advocated a view of quality improvement in medicine that rests not on fear but on aspiration, quality improvement begins with the question, "In what ways would I like to improve?"[2] To answer this question, physicians first need to know how they compare with their colleagues by specialty, age, geographical area, practice size, practice type, and a host of other variables that make the data they review and the message they receive about nonclinical office risk management efforts relevant to their practice.

The PA/QI program gathers those data from practicing physicians and presents them to participants in a form that enables them to measure with precision their performance in relation to their peers. At that point, change in nonclinical practice and behavior patterns becomes a matter of informed choice. To date, OMA's findings document that, given the choice, participants have chosen to make and continue to support practice changes that decrease in-office claims exposure. It is also relevant that it is their professional association—not a regulatory body, liability insurer, or third-party payer—that provides these data as a member service in a nondemanding and nonpunitive way.

Risk Management Messages Must Offer Reasonable Solutions

Program participants receive the AMA/SSMLP's publication entitled *Risk Management Principles & Commentaries for the Medical Office (Ps and Cs)*. This 31-page document is a succinct compilation of the prevailing wisdom, with rationales, on nonclinical risk management issues in the office environment. It is an important tool in the PA/QI program, where its frequent use as a resource for both physicians and their employees is encouraged.

The Oregon Medical Association conducted and videotaped interviews with sitting trial judges and defense attorneys. They were asked to comment on many questions from the self-assessment survey in terms of whether failure to adhere to the advice contained in the *Principles & Commentaries* materially affected the outcome of a malpractice claim. Oregon's PA/QI participants can watch the interviews while preparing for the home-study course. Hearing a judge or defense lawyer give case examples of how claims are compromised by specific nonclinical practices or behaviors has been seen as very helpful by the participants. State pilot sites are being encouraged to provide their participants with similar material as may be appropriate for their locales.

Any Successful Program Must Have Specialty-Specific Elements

Loss-prevention issues in the medical office are largely non–specialty-specific, insofar as the focus is on communications and administrative systems rather than the clinical practice of medicine. Hence, the PA/QI self-assessment survey shown in figure 15-1 is a "core questionnaire" believed to be relevant to all office-based practitioners. However, each specialty approaches some nonclinical practice matters in a slightly different fashion. Therefore, specialty-specific questions are under development to be added to the core questionnaire.

The home-study course segment of PA/QI uses specialty-specific case histories, primarily to provide a more effective learning experience. The loss-prevention issues may be the same across specialties, but the impact on participants is enhanced when the examples used look most like their own practice. In addition, specialty-specific issues can be addressed.

☐ Findings Concerning PA/QI's Three Integrated Elements

Data from the Oregon experience as of mid-1991 have been tabulated and evaluated. The results of this analysis of more than 1,400 surveys provide a snapshot of PA/QI program participants and their risk management experience.

Self-Assessment Survey Results

The following results were compiled from the self-assessment survey:

- Demographic data:
  —*Gender:* Male participant/physicians (85.5 percent) substantially outnumber female participant/physicians
  —*Practice type:* Participating physicians practice in group settings (49.2 percent) more frequently than either their office-sharing (18.5 percent) or their solo-practice (32.2 percent) counterparts.
  —*Specialty:* A broad spectrum of specialties is represented (48 to date). Most frequently represented are internists (19.38 percent), family physicians (14.50 percent), ophthalmologists (7.28 percent), obstetrician/gynecologists (6.01 percent), surgeons (5.80 percent), and pediatricians (5.73 percent).
  —*Age:* Participants range in age from 29 to 82 years. Solo practitioners are slightly older (50.0 years) than those who share offices (46.0 years) or practice in groups (45.0 years).
- Claim frequency and severity data:
  —*Claims per physician:* The number of claims per participating physician range from 0 (59.6 percent) to 11 (.07 percent). Physicians with one claim represent 23.4 percent of the sample.
  —*Office type:* Although solo-practice physicians represent 32.2 percent of the current survey sample, they account for 36.2 percent of the claims and 49.6 percent of the dollars paid. As a result, OMA may place special emphasis on the risk management needs of the solo practitioner. This percentage imbalance will be investigated further.
  —*Specialty:* Do certain specialties have a frequency of claims that is disproportionate to their participation in the SAS data base? For the most part, results based on some 1,400 surveys tend to confirm common beliefs concerning "high-risk" and "low-risk" specialties. Although obstetricians represent only 6.01 percent of the participants, they have 11.96 percent of the claims and are responsible for 20.47 percent of the indemnity paid. Ophthalmologists, on the other hand, represent 7.28 percent of the survey participants but account for only 3.82 percent of the claims and 1.32 percent of the dollars paid. Some findings deserve further study. For instance, dermatologists represent 2.9 percent of the participants and have only 1.67 percent of the claims. However, their claims account for 4.01 percent of the dollars paid. Surgeons (5.80 percent), on the other hand, have a claim frequency maldistribution (9.31 percent of all claims) but a relatively low claim severity (3.91 percent of all dollars paid).
- Aggregate risk management behavior profiles:
  —*Correlation:* The SAS is divided into 13 sections. The OMA found that each section of the SAS is highly correlated statistically with every other section. The data suggest that physicians who engage in one type of risk management activity are likely to engage in others. For example, those physicians practicing risk management behaviors in their record documentation habits were more likely to have adequate liability control measures in other parts of their clinical

practice. This suggests that physicians are amenable to receiving information about risk management that may touch on multiple areas of their practices.

—*Effects of age on behavior:* Older physicians are statistically more likely to perform certain risk management behaviors than their younger colleagues. Perhaps as physicians mature in practice they compensate for a loss of stamina, drive, skills, or interest by adopting defensive practices of a nonclinical nature. Again, OMA will investigate this finding further. It may dictate a different approach to doing risk management education with younger physicians.

Home-Study Course Results

Reaction to the course has been enthusiastic and supportive. Participants took between two and one-half and five hours to complete it. Seventy-five percent of the participants felt that the home-study course was well organized and easy to use. Eighty-three percent felt that completing the home-study course helped them in their practices. Following are some representative comments on this subject:

- "The course brings to attention what the recurring issues really are and how these issues may put one at risk."
- "It reinforces what I already know, but doesn't force me to do it."
- "Excellent job. I can see every one of my partners and me in those scenarios."
- "I noted correctable parallels between some of the portrayed physicians and my own personality and practice."

A committee of OMA physicians is currently reviewing every evaluation of the home-study course, and revisions are under way. More medical record excerpts will be added as well as other slight changes suggested by participants' comments.

On-Site Visit Results

The most striking conclusion reached from the on-site visits conducted to date is that physicians made substantial, yet very different, changes to their practices and in their behaviors following completion of both the SAS and the home-study course. Most of the process changes occurred following completion of the SAS. Quite clearly, the SAS focuses predominantly on process issues. According to participants, they were stimulated to make a number of process-oriented changes in response to their "no" answers on the SAS. Frequently, however, behavior changes were made by physicians only after completion of the home-study course. For them, seeing an association between a behavior they could identify with and an actual malpractice claim was enough to cause a serious reevaluation of their behaviors toward patients, colleagues, or coworkers.

A number of changes occurred only after the on-site visit took place. Most participants attributed this to the fact that until they were able to speak face-to-face with surveyors, they remained unconvinced that these changes were appropriate. Some physicians were persuaded by a review of their individual assessment report. Others made changes after receiving detailed explanations from the surveyors.

☐ AMA/SSMLP Pilot Project

The AMA/Specialty Society Medical Liability Project and state medical associations and liability insurers in eight additional states will be testing the effectiveness of the PA/QI program during the next two years.

An important benefit of the expanded pilot project will be the establishment of a national registry of PA/QI self-assessment data. This registry will be based in Illinois, where peer review data confidentiality is protected from disclosure by a strong state statute, and it will process the questionnaires received from all PA/QI physician participants. It is a goal of the project to have the PA/QI registry operational by mid-1992. By the end of 1992, at least 250 responses from each pilot site will have been collected and tabulated. In this way, the first accurate national data on nonclinical risk management behaviors and practices tabulated by specialty, gender, age, practice type, and malpractice claims experience will be available in aggregate for further study and discussion.

☐ Conclusion

Preliminary results of the PA/QI project in Oregon are promising. Physicians have expressed a strong desire for information about how to improve their nonclinical risk management activities in the medical office. The PA/QI project appears to address this need. It brings together for the first time three proven educational methods—self-assessment, home study, and comparative feedback—that allow the participants to focus on their individual practices while at the same time drawing from statewide experience. Testing of the PA/QI project on a national basis will occur through the end of 1993. It is hoped that the results from the eight additional state pilot sites will demonstrate that PA/QI is a workable educational model for improving the quality of patient care and reducing the frequency and severity of claims arising out of treatment of patients in the medical office.

The PA/QI program is a unique example of how physicians can provide their colleagues with a process that they can use to (1) assess their own quality from a risk management perspective, and (2) help them make practice changes that will improve the quality of patient care, minimize patient injury, or reduce the risk of malpractice litigation.

☐ References

1. Frisch, P. Risk Assessment and Management Program. In: P. L. Spath, editor. *Innovations in Health Care Quality Measurement*. Chicago: American Hospital Publishing, 1989.

2. Berwick, D. M., Godfrey, A. B., and Roessner, J. *Curing Health Care: New Strategies for Quality Improvement*. San Francisco: Jossey-Bass, 1990, pp. 48–49.

Chapter 16

Quality Care Review Program

Barbara Toeppen-Sprigg, M.D., and Dewey C. Scheid, M.D.

Throughout the past 29 years, there has been considerable progress made in the development of the theory and practice of health care quality management. Yet to date, most applications of quality management theory have occurred in hospitals, whereas the bulk of the medical care in the United States occurs in the offices of primary care physicians, many of whom have yet to initiate formal quality review programs.

Since 1988, the Ohio Academy of Family Physicians (OAFP) has sponsored, through its quality assessment committee, an office-based quality review program evaluating the clinical and administrative aspects of primary care. The quality care review program was initiated to assist motivated physicians in their quest to provide excellent care through a periodic audit process that allows for annual assessments of a physician's individual performance. Participants in this project are offered the opportunity to compare their practices with those of their peers.

☐ The Quality Care Review Program

Members of the specialty of family practice are aware of the need to remain current in medical information, and their professional organizations have reflected this concern. The American Board of Family Practice was the first to require recertification of members on a seven-year cycle.[1] Part of this recertification process requires that members abstract information from actual patient charts from their offices and compare their patient care practices with standards established by the American Board of Family Practice.

The OAFP felt that family physicians also needed a longitudinal process of review. The quality care review program was established and directed toward self-assessment and self-education, providing benefits to patient care that go beyond the board recertification process. The quality care review program was also established to help physicians meet future regulatory office-based quality review mandates that might be imposed on the medical profession. By designing quality review models, the OAFP felt confident it could influence the development of practice policies that would enhance primary health care delivery. It was felt that the administrative aspects of medical care are just as important as the clinical components. Therefore, methods for evaluating the quality of clinic office practices and the patient management elements receive equal attention in the quality review process.

Participants

Initial funding for the quality care review program was provided by the OAFP, but the subscriptions paid by participants after the start of the program have covered the costs over the first four years with minor additional support. The target population for the quality care review program is intended to be family physicians. A review of subscribers in 1990 indicated that 93.6 percent of participants identified themselves as family physicians, with 89.7 percent of the subscribers being board certified.[2] Forty-seven percent of the participants describe themselves as sole practitioners; an additional 22 percent report being in small group practices of three or fewer physicians. Approximately 47 percent of the participants practice in cities with populations of less than 10,000. As of the 1990 cycle, there were a total of 425 program subscribers from 14 states. Only 24.7 percent of the participants were from Ohio.

Review Topics

The review topics included in the quality assessment project are selected by the quality assessment committee of the OAFP. Medical topics for clinical reviews are divided among acute illness, chronic illness, and asymptomatic screening. The clinical reviews are created by family practice residencies throughout the state of Ohio. Each residency selected by the medical directors is given the clinical question to be addressed by the review. The responsible faculty, with the assistance of the residents, researches the clinical topic, performing literature reviews, selecting the review criteria, and supplying reference documentation for each selected criterion. The medical directors edit the criteria and references to fit the format and style of the overall program. Administrative reviews are designed by the medical directors with the assistance of private physicians and other appropriate professionals such as practice managers and financial advisers.

The quality care review program does little to measure the *effectiveness* of patient care. The criteria may reflect how well a physician cares for patients with fairly well-defined diseases, but they do not measure diagnostic accuracy. The quality care review studies also do not attempt to measure outcomes. The administrative criteria evaluate the organization and efficiency of the office, and in some cases are reflective of patient outcomes, but not in direct relation to the medical care provided by the physician.

☐ Program Design

Each quarter, the subscriber receives a packet of two sets of criteria—one clinical and one administrative—for a particular topic.

Clinical Review

The clinical review consists of five major criteria (see figure 16-1) for the review of a medical question, such as "Is the initial evaluation of a patient with acute low back pain appropriate?" Other examples of clinical reviews include well-infant care, hypertension evaluation, breast cancer screening, and medical care of diabetes mellitus. The clinical review usually requires data collection from 10 records. Participants indicate whether or not each of the five criteria is met. For each criterion that is not met, the participants indicate who is responsible for the variance—physician, staff, or patient. Included in the packet of criteria is a set of references that provide background information and substantiation for each criterion in the study. Of those surveyed, 87.1 percent thought

Figure 16-1. Clinical Study Criteria

Quality Care Review #201

The Question: Is the initial evaluation of a patient with acute low back pain appropriate?
(10 records to be reviewed)

Chart Selection: Select 10 charts of patients of any age who have had an appointment for acute low back pain within the past five years.

Objective Criteria:

1. The history must include:

   a. Onset and duration of symptoms
   b. Location and radiation of pain
   c. Previous history of back pain [Ref. #1, #4, #5, #12]

2. The history must include the presence or absence of neurological complaints. [Ref. #6, #13]

3. The physical examination must include:

   a. Location of tenderness
   b. Back flexibility
   c. Straight leg raising [Ref. #7, #8, #10]

4. The physical examination must include the presence or absence of neurological findings [Ref. #9]

5. Radiographic evaluation (or referral) must be done in the presence of:

   a. History of a traumatic injury
   b. Suspicion of a compression fracture, malignancy, or infection
   c. Significant neurological deficit such as cauda equina syndrome [Ref. #2, #3, #11]

Procedure:

1. Review the chart and record the findings on the evaluation form.

2. Complete the summary form and return to *Quality Care Review* by the deadline.

Due Date: _____

these references were informative, and 87.6 percent thought the references did a good job of supporting the objective criteria. The individual chart review results are recorded on a standard evaluation form (figure 16-2). Data from each evaluation form are then summarized and transferred to a study summary form (figure 16-3), which is to be returned to the quality care review program within six weeks.

Administrative Review

The administrative review portion of the study series consists of a variable number of criteria for evaluation of topics, such as "Does your office laboratory give reliable results?" Other topics of administrative review include telephone availability, medical record keeping, practice accessibility, and physician–patient communication. An evaluation form is provided for the administrative review, and study participants indicate whether or not criteria are met. References are not routinely provided with the administrative reviews. As with the clinical review, the results are transferred to a summary form and returned within six weeks.

☐ Principles of the Study

The basic tenet of the program is that the most effective review is self-review. The physician is responsible for comparing chart records to the audit criteria, summing the results, using the information gleaned to assess performance, stating the changes that

Figure 16-2. Review Evaluation Form

Medical Care

PATIENT IDENTITY*	CRITERIA	MET	NOT MET PATIENT	NOT MET STAFF	NOT MET PHYSICIAN	COMMENTS
————	1					
	2					
	3					
	4					
	5					
————	1					
	2					
	3					
	4					
	5					
————	1					
	2					
	3					
	4					
	5					
————	1					
	2					
	3					
	4					
	5					
————	1					
	2					
	3					
	4					
	5					

NOTES:

*FOR YOUR USE ONLY

need to be made as a result of the audit, and planning follow-up. This process is facilitated by providing evaluation and summary forms with each review. Although the physician is responsible for the performance of the review, in some cases office staff participate, especially in the administrative reviews. A statement as to who actually participated in the review is not requested, so little is known regarding the level of office staff participation. A recent subscriber survey revealed a mean of 3.1 hours being spent on each review.

The objective criteria used to review medical care and administrative performance evaluate the process of health care delivery by determining compliance with specific components of care for selected patients with acute illness or chronic illness, or during

Figure 16-3. Review Summary Form

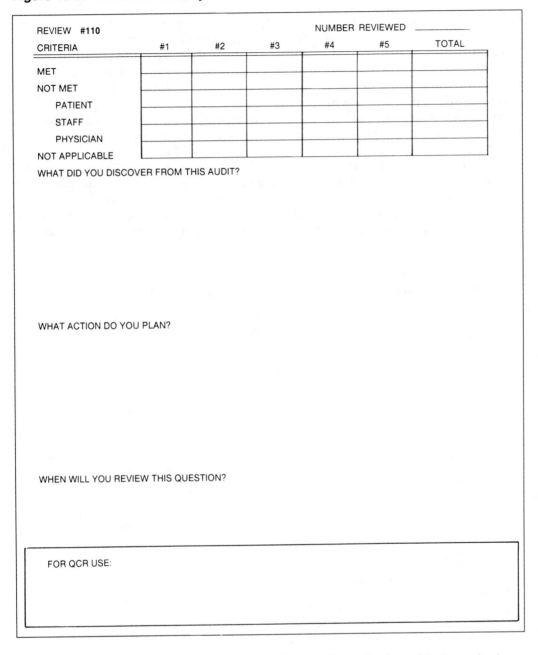

REVIEW #110   NUMBER REVIEWED _____

CRITERIA	#1	#2	#3	#4	#5	TOTAL
MET						
NOT MET						
PATIENT						
STAFF						
PHYSICIAN						
NOT APPLICABLE						

WHAT DID YOU DISCOVER FROM THIS AUDIT?

WHAT ACTION DO YOU PLAN?

WHEN WILL YOU REVIEW THIS QUESTION?

FOR QCR USE:

asymptomatic screening. Although each study includes only five objective criteria, many criteria consist of subcomponents like the objective criteria in the example of acute low back pain (figure 16-1). Participants are asked to decide whether or not the overall criteria were met even though one or more of the subcriteria may be missing. Only 25.8 percent of surveyed participants favored scoring the individual components of more complex criteria. For this reason, the quality care review program limits most studies to five major objective criteria combined with limited chart review. Unfortunately, this constraint allows for an evaluation of only a sample of the care provided, but a more comprehensive review is avoided in order to control the participant's record review time requirements. Even with imposed restrictions on the number of criteria in each study, chart review currently requires a bigger time commitment than 74.4 percent of surveyed subscribers wish to spend.

☐ Communication and Feedback

Interaction between subscribers and study editors is facilitated by two mechanisms. The first is communication coming from the subscriber to the study editors. Each study summary form (figure 16-3) has a space for comments at the bottom, and subscribers are encouraged to critique the review topics and corresponding criteria. The second is feedback from the study editors to the subscribers. At the end of each series, the comparative report includes a brief commentary on the general performance of the enrollment group, responses to participant comments and questions, and information about other issues in quality assurance. The cycle of one complete quality assurance project is shown in figure 16-4.

At the end of each study series, which lasts one year (one packet of reviews per quarter—each packet containing a clinical study and an administrative study), a report is sent to the physician/subscriber comparing his or her individual performance with that of all same-series study participants (figure 16-5). Comparisons are reported by the percentage of all cases meeting the criteria for each of the eight reviews during the same cycle.

Figure 16-4.   Cycle of One Complete Quality Assurance Project

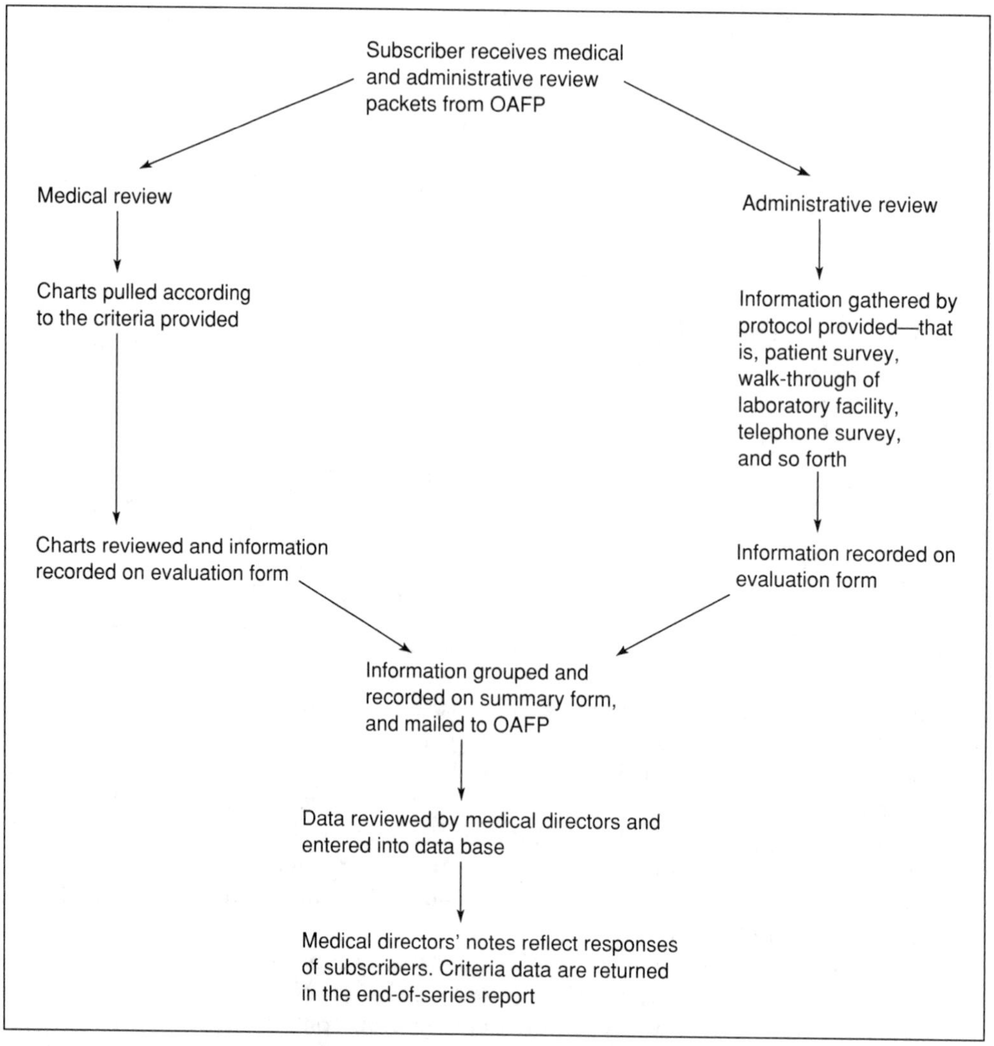

Figure 16-5. Report of Comparison Data for One Series of Quality Care Review

This certifies that physician #266 has participated in the 1989–90 OAFP Quality Care Review, which has been approved for 15 hours of prescribed credit by the American Academy of Family Physicians. Scoring shows the percentage of cases meeting the study criteria for each topic.

Summary of Your Returns
Confidential

Quality Care Review Study Number and Topic		Criterion No. 1	Criterion No. 2	Criterion No. 3	Criterion No. 4	Criterion No. 5
#101 Care for Year-Old Child						
	Your Score	20	80	10	60	80
	Peer Score	70.5	83	48	85	79
#102 Telephone Availability						
	Your Score	90	100	75	80	80
	Peer Score	92	89	91	92	85
#103 Evaluation of Hypertension						
	Your Score	45	0	36	36	100
	Peer Score	74	44	92	70	89
#104 Adequate Medical Records						
	Your Score	100	100	100	100	95
	Peer Score	94	84	79	94	99
#105 Sore Throat/Rheumatic Fever						
	Your Score	80	70	90	30	50
	Peer Score	91	63	82	84	89
#106 Availability of Medical Services						
	Your Score	72	84	92	96	100
	Peer Score	93	82	94	94	97
#107 Appropriate Screening for Breast Lesions						
	Your Score	20	50	0	20	90
	Peer Score	78	78	65	80	95
#108 Physician–Patient Communication						
	Your Score	100	100	40	90	100
	Peer Score	97	91	73	87	90

No report of summary data or physician-specific results is made to any regulatory or credentialing agency, but continuing medical education (CME) credit offered by the American Academy of Family Practice can be earned by the study participant. Included with the review feedback is a brief educational article related to quality assurance, such as "How to Generate an Office-Based Quality Assurance Log." The articles selected by the quality care review program staff to distribute with the study feedback are designed to enhance the knowledge of physicians and office staff in the basic principles of outpatient quality assessment and improvement.

The quality care review program is administered through the OAFP headquarters staff, who are responsible for marketing, publication, and distribution, as well as for solution of subscriber problems. Data from each summary form received from the subscribers are entered into a personal computer. Through use of the data-base package Q & A™, reports are generated and shared with the subscribers at the end of the review series. Most of the cost of the quality care review is ascribed to this central information system support and reporting function. The annual charge for participation is $110 for members of the American Academy of Family Practice and $140 for nonmembers. This yearly fee covers the cost of four review packets and the comparative report that is produced and shared with the subscribers at the end of each study series. Physicians interested in participating in the quality review project can obtain more information by contacting the Quality Care Review Program, Ohio Academy of Family Practice, 4075 North High Street, Columbus, OH 43214-3296; 614/267-7867.

☐ Program Results and Future Plans

This is the fourth year of the quality care review project, and work is beginning on the 500 series topics. It has been an educational process for the study developers as well as the participants. A challenge has been to balance the comprehensiveness of reviews with the time constraints and expectations for degree of complexity of the participants. However, a survey of participants completed in 1990 showed that 90 percent of the subscribers feel that the studies' objective criteria are relevant to basic quality care, and 75 percent of the subscribers are reportedly satisfied with the quantity of chart review required. Forty-seven percent believe the quality care review studies have improved their medical care; 33 percent are undecided.

Plans are in the works to expand the review packets to include not just topic criteria lists but also clinical algorithms that would permit evaluation of diagnostic decision making. Although this enhancement will make the reviews more difficult to design and will require different computer software to report results to subscribers, the quality care review medical directors agree this is a worthwhile goal. As developments in medical outcome research become available, the program will integrate this information into future reviews. The quality care review program would also like to investigate why variations of clinical practice occur and to analyze the features that account for differences in expert recommendation and routine clinical practice.

☐ Conclusion

The quality care review program has made a significant contribution to the practice of quality assessment and improvement in private physician practice. Through the development of a quick and simple method of longitudinal practice review that encourages individual primary care physicians to evaluate themselves in comparison to peers, the medical community moves closer to the goal of comprehensive quality management. The basic premise of the quality care review program—that self-review is the best quality improvement motivator—remains as constant today as when the program was originated.

☐ References

1. American Board of Family Practice. *Directory of Diplomates: 1991.* Lexington, KY: ABFP, 1991, p. ix.

2. Report to Quality Assessment Committee. Ohio Academy of Family Physicians, Apr. 7, 1990, Akron, OH, p. 3.